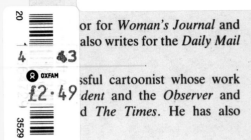
or for *Woman's Journal* and
also writes for the *Daily Mail*

ssful cartoonist whose work
dent and the *Observer* and
d *The Times*. He has also

Dr Paul Clayton is the health editor of ... resident doctor for UK Living. He ... and Marie Claire.

Jonathan Pugh is a highly successful ... appears regularly in the Independent ... occasionally in the Guardian and ... illustrated a number of books.

STOP COUNTING SHEEP

Self help for Insomnia

Dr Paul Clayton

HEADLINE

First published in 1994
by HEADLINE BOOK PUBLISHING

10 9 8 7 6 5 4 3 2 1

ISBN 0 7472 4336 0

Typeset by
Letterpart Limited, Reigate, Surrey

Printed and bound in Great Britain by
HarperCollins Manufacturing, Glasgow

HEADLINE BOOK PUBLISHING
A division of Hodder Headline PLC
Headline House
79 Great Titchfield Street
London W1P 7FN

Contents

1. Sleep – who needs it?   1
2. What do you do when you can't sleep?   9
3. Why sleep goes wrong   13
4. Nightmares and night terrors   18
5. Snoring   22
6. Categories of insomnia – which one are you?   27
7. Tired all the time   31
8. Sleep and health   36
9. Duration of insomnia: is this you?   39
10. Special groups: children, adolescents and the
    elderly   45
11. An insomniac's progress through the medical
    system   50
12. Sleeping pills   58
13. The better sleep programme   63
14. Melatonin   70
15. Yet more remedies   72
16. Eat to sleep   78
17. Meal timing   85
18. Sex and sleep   89
19. Pain prevention   97
20. Anxiety reduction   102
21. Panic attacks   105
22. Coping with seasonal insomnia   109

23. Allergies and asthma   114
24. Cold wars – sleeping through the sneezes   116
25. General health and sleep   120
26. Acupuncture and acupressure   126
27. Massage and oils   131
28. Geopathic stress   136
29. Sleep diary   142
30. Useful contacts   143
31. Brain machines   147
     Index   149

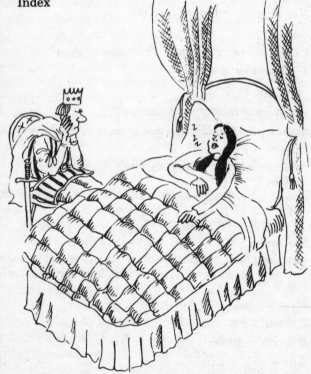

HOW MUCH SLEEP DO WE NEED ?

CHAPTER 1

Sleep – who needs it?

You're wide awake – tossing and turning – and the clock tells you it's that seemingly interminable hour of 3 a.m. Five more hours like this, and you will have to get up and start the day. You crave oblivion, but your mind seems more concerned with that unpaid gas bill than hazy lazy images of woolly sheep in lush pastures. It's a nightmare, isn't it? OK, that's a bit of a misnomer, since you would probably welcome a real 'X' certificate nightmare if it involved some snoozing beforehand – but let's face it, insomnia is no joke. When you're in this state, it seems as if the world and his wife are safely tucked up in bed, drifting luxuriously into glorious slumberland, and, lucky things, without the slightest of difficulties.

Have you noticed how good insomniacs are at self torture? When I suffered from serial bouts of sleeplessness, some demon would compel me to get up and look out of the window, and the mere sight of all those drawn curtains down the road concealing cosy bedrooms and sleeping bodies was enough to make me feel completely enraged and very lonely indeed. In this mood, I was convinced the whole globe shared the same time zone – and even in the depths of Australia there would be cities and towns and streets heaving gently to the rhythm of comforting snoozing!

I also thought I would go mad without a decent few hours' worth of restorative kip. But rest assured, lack of sleep does not drive you mad – nor do we need as much sleep as we think. Sleep deprivation doesn't necessarily make you ill, although there is evidence that a chronic shortfall of sleep will eventually impair the functioning of the immune system, which will increase your risk of catching coughs, colds and other bugs.

WHAT CAUSES INSOMNIA?

Insomnia does not seem to correspond to a type of employment (or unemployment); although night work and shift work have a tendency to increase the risk of someone developing sleeping problems. But what does matter, more than anything else, is how stressed you are. Stress is the single most common cause of poor sleep, and later I will suggest ways of dealing with this prevalent problem.

Everyone knows what it feels like to be under stress. Sense of humour is one of the first things to go, closely followed by patience, tolerance and temper. Then there's the churning stomach, the racing heart, and the feelings of helplessness or even depression. But central to all of this, and a key factor in making all of the other symptoms worse, is insomnia. Scratch an insomniac, and you'll find in most cases a man or a woman under stress.

At the risk of offending the politically correct brigade, men and women experience stress from rather different sources. Men, as you might have guessed, worry and fret themselves mostly about work. Women, on the other hand, relate most of their stress to personal life, emotional issues and family problems. But in both cases, the problem boils down to a common denominator: too much stress leaves the victim keyed up, and unable to relax or switch off.

Other common causes of insomnia include certain foods and drinks, especially if consumed late in the evening; and uncomfortable or unsuitable sleeping arrangements. A surprising number of insomniacs blame it on a partner with a bad snoring habit; and, although it's hard to believe, others can't get off to sleep because they're all tense and worried about not being able to get off to sleep – or oversleeping in the morning.

THE EXTREMES OF SLEEP DEPRIVATION

In the longest studies of sleep deprivation, where the unfortunate subjects were kept awake under controlled conditions for periods of up to ten days, a number of neurophysiological changes were seen. Apart from tiredness, which was hardly surprising, the experimenters recorded trembling of the eyes and hands, and increased irritability. In addition, the subjects did less well in tests measuring vigilance, rapidity of response, and judgement. Interestingly, the sense of touch was increased in some but not all the victims, sorry, experimental subjects.

Amazingly, the subjects were still fairly alert in the mornings, but their performance and their tempers deteriorated in the small hours. This pattern reflected the normal drive to wake in the morning and sleep at night.

The effects of sleep deprivation have also been studied under battlefield conditions. Troops chronically short of sleep can still function perfectly well during moments of crisis, such as an attack or an exchange of gunfire – the rush of adrenalin is enough to keep body and soul ticking over for a while. But the same soldiers will forget the routines of filling their water bottles, petrol tanks or ammunition clips, with dangerous and often fatal results.

Apart from the ability to concentrate, the ability to make measured decisions is also affected. This is probably more or less what you'd expect, and is well known to the business community who play one-upmanship games by scheduling meetings to put the other side at a disadvantage. Catching the other team just off the red-eye night flight is an old tactic, as is scheduling meetings at a time when the opposition would normally be tucked up in bed. This is the time to go in hard, knowing that their negotiating skills and stamina are at a low point. (The Gestapo used a similar technique, hauling suspects out of bed in the small hours of the morning when they knew their victims would show least resistance.)

HOW MUCH SLEEP DO WE NEED?

The reason why we're more alert at specific times during the day, and experience definite lulls at others, and why we prefer to sleep at certain times but remain bafflingly awake at other periods, is to do with the 24-hour alarm clock built into our brains.

Bats require an astonishing 19 hours of sleep out of the 24, and cats, as many of you already suspect, sleep (and cat-nap) up to 15 hours a day. This makes our 8 hours look quite reasonable – until you consider the cow, which gets by with 4 hours, and the horse, which requires only 3 hours.

But not everybody insists on the statutory 8 hours. Some boast of managing on as little as 3 or 4 hours. Many teenagers seem to be able to sleep quite happily for up to 15 hours a day (although in some cases this may be a symptom of a depressive illness). Einstein was a well-known long sleeper. At the other end of the scale, Voltaire only needed 3 hours of sleep a night, and both Napoleon and Churchill were known to be very short sleepers.

On a somewhat lesser scale, Margaret Thatcher used to make a point of her ability to work a 20-hour day, a claim designed to impress her male colleagues – but how does she fill the empty hours between midnight and dawn now that she's safely out of office? What is a normal amount of sleep, and what is necessary?

In the Western world, the majority (about 60 per cent) of the population regularly sleeps between 6½ and 8½ hours each night. That leaves 40 per cent, who split into two more or less equal groups; the long sleepers, who put in more than 8½ hours, and the short sleepers, who get by on less than 6½. But the range is wider than this, because quite a few (and not a few captains of industry and politics) require less than 5 hours.

Quite apart from personal proclivities, sleep requirements vary with age. Babies need about 15 hours of sleep out of the

24; adults of between 20 and 60 years need an average of about 7 hours; and the over-65s need a bit less, about 6½ hours.

If you consider that the latter age group may well be taking naps during the day, which reduce the need for night-time sleep, yet still going to bed at the same time as before, then it's no surprise that they find it is taking a bit longer to get to sleep, and that they wake more often during the night. This pattern, although it is pretty normal, in the sense that it happens to nearly everybody, is often interpreted as insomnia. But how insomniac is the insomniac?

Most people overestimate the time they spend lying awake by a factor of as much as three, so it is difficult to judge accurately, without making a sleep diary (see Appendix 1) or relying on a partner to note down the details. Even so, lying awake in a dark bedroom can be boring, and it can allow the mind to dwell on concerns and worries.

DIFFERENT KINDS OF SLEEP

When we go to bed and fall asleep we are not aware of the different stages of sleep that our brains must go through to reap the full benefit of a good night's sleep. Let's take a look at these.

Awake in bed
We all know what it feels like to be awake. We're conscious, aware of our surroundings, and of what we're thinking. We are intermittently aware also of feelings such as hunger, thirst, irritation and all the other human emotions; and as the brain processes all these thoughts and feelings, the millions of nerve cells fire, and keep on firing, producing irregular, sharp little waves of electric current that ripple across the surface of the brain. These can be monitored by a device known as an electroencephalograph.

Sleep states

Stage 1

The first and lightest of the sleep stages, or in layperson's terms, drowsiness. It is the gateway between wakefulness and true sleep; the subject is easily roused, and intrusive sounds or lights are more likely to be disturbing during this stage than later in the cycle, when the sleeper has descended into the deeper stages of sleep. But already the body has begun to change; our muscles begin to relax, the brow unfurrows; and as sleep continues to knit up the ravelled sleeve of care, heart rate, blood pressure, and the digestive processes all begin to wind down for the night.

Meanwhile, back in the brain, things have also begun to slow down for the night. Slower waves begin to increase; you'll see them not only in Stage 1 sleepers, but also in meditators, people in hypnotic trances, and watchers of TV soap operas. This stage doesn't occupy much time; you're on your way down, and within 2–10 minutes you enter . . .

Stage 2

Stage 2 is a bit of a mixture – the brain is by this stage switching between medium slow waves and slow waves. As it does, we drift between light sleep and deep unconsciousness. It's a gentle oceanic swell, and lasts for nearly half of our sleeping time. Then, after a period in Stage 2, somewhere in the brain a relay clicks open, and we drift effortlessly down into . . .

Stage 3

Which is, like Stage 1, a sort of airlock. You don't stay long in Stage 3, but you have to go through it to get to Stage 4. As the descent through Stage 3 continues, the brain waves become progressively slower. Within a few minutes you leave Stage 3 and step out on the ocean floor.

Stage 4
This is the deepest form of sleep. Sluggish waves of electrical pulses move over the surface of the brain, and we're out for the count. In an average night we'll spend between 35 and 50 minutes here, in 4 or 5 bouts of around ten minutes each. The total length of time in Stage 4 diminishes with age, although there are exceptions to this rule.

Rapid eye movement or REM sleep
Periods of REM sleep are almost always preceded by periods of non-REM sleep, where the brain waves get progressively larger and slower. Then, over at the electroencephalograph, the sleep scientist will suddenly hear the polygraph pens dancing to a different rhythm. The pens monitoring bodily movement stop, and the physical activity trace runs flat along the bottom of the graph; but the pens that record brain cell activity burst into frantic life, scratching wildly across the paper, and telling us that a dream has begun.

When the brain switches to REM sleep, a number of odd things happen. Firstly, the EEG suddenly changes over to something that resembles an awake or lightly dozing brain – although sleepers are very difficult to arouse during REM sleep. The sleeper experiences visual dreams, in black and white or colour, often complete with sound and even touch; and the eyes move about rapidly, as if following some action, presumably the imagery in the dream. Pulse and breathing rates quicken and the amount of electrical activity in the muscles drops to almost zero.

In a typical night, the sleeper regularly moves through the cycles of sleep, from 1 to 4, then from 4 back to 1. From Stage 1 he or she often flips into REM sleep, before beginning the descent once again towards Stage 4. In a typical night the sleeper will move through the entire cycle some 4 or 5 times.

The length of the cycle varies between different individuals, between 80 and 120 minutes; but in any individual, the cycle is of fixed length, constituting a sort of sleep fingerprint. However, the amount of time spent in each stage of

7

sleep varies through the night.

When you first fall asleep, the brain descends through Stages 1 and 2, and into Stages 3 and 4 very rapidly, and spends as much as an hour in deep sleep. During this part of the night the sleeper is much harder to wake. The REM period that follows, the first of the night, is usually very short. Later cycles have less deep sleep, but more REM sleep. By the last cycle before waking, the brain spends most of the cycle, as much as a whole hour, in REM; and it is dream material from this REM period which is most likely to be recalled after waking.

The total time spent in REM sleep is about 25 per cent of the sleeping time. In other words, we spend between 1½ and 2 hours dreaming every night – so there's a lot more to our dream lives than we remember. And some people dream more than others; long sleepers spend more time in REM than short sleepers, because long sleepers have more cycles, and the late cycles have more REM. Despite this, there is no correlation between long sleeping and creativity.

CHAPTER 2

What do you do when you can't sleep?

Still hopelessly wide awake? So what do you do? Many insomniacs eventually give up the struggle, stop worrying about not sleeping and get up and try to do something active to take their minds off the problem. They go to the kitchen to make a drink, or dive into the bedside book. There's always the radio, and even the television if you don't mind a diet of Open University programmes, mixed with the compulsively awful ITV night viewing. Some go for a walk, which might be OK in more select neighbourhoods but is pretty darn hazardous if you live in an inner urban area. Tidier souls opt for housework, getting through piles of dirty dishes, ironing, or even knitting. A few might start work on a novel; and some, inadvisably, reach for the sleeping tablets, which, if taken too late at night, will leave you with a drug-induced hangover the next morning.

Surprisingly, however, the vast majority of insomniacs do not go to their doctor for help. In fact, surveys suggest that for every patient who does go to the doctor, there are another 256 who don't. One reason for their lack of enthusiasm is that they worry that the doctor will give them sleeping pills, which will result in their becoming addicted.

These fears are not entirely groundless, because although most doctors are now very careful about prescribing this sort of medication, medical enthusiasm for the benzodiazepines (the commonest form of sleeping pill) in the sixties and seventies created large numbers of addicts. The Council for Involuntary Tranquilliser Addiction, CITA, based in

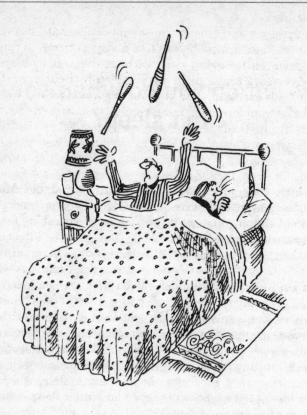

WHAT DO YOU DO WHEN YOU CAN'T SLEEP

Liverpool, estimates that there are nearly 2,000,000 Britons still addicted to sleeping pills – a figure which has not declined much over the last decade or so, suggesting that for many the tranquilliser habit is just too difficult to break.

SARAH'S STORY

'I've always slept badly – even as a little girl, and unbelievably I was prescribed sleeping pills and valium when I was still only in my early teens. There's no doubt that I got very reliant on these drugs – it was like a vicious circle, in that I was convinced I couldn't sleep without them. It took me a good five years to cut them out completely. I cut down the dosage, and eventually did without them altogether. Yes, I still suffer from insomnia, but recently I've been trying some alternative methods which have really helped. Herbal teas like vervain and camomile with honey have a very calming effect; I also have a slow relaxing bath before bedtime. And if I still can't sleep, I try changing my attitude to sleeplessness. Previously I would fret about feeling tired the next day – now I try and enjoy the feeling of being warm and cosy in bed, and I concentrate on all the good things going on in my life, rather than the negative things. I'm sure this helps give me relaxation, if not always fully fledged sleep.'

More on Sarah's self help later. But as for many other poor sleepers, they are simply convinced that their doctor wouldn't be able to help much, and that sleeplessness is a problem that they just have to live with. This isn't entirely true, because in many cases the doctor can help. This might just be a reassurance that it doesn't really matter if you don't sleep well; or it might be a prescription of sleeping pills with advice on how to take them without becoming dependent on them. Some patients appreciate being sent to a specialist – but the truth is that what doctors are best at is treating those cases of insomnia caused by underlying illness. This is what doctors are trained to do, and in this sub-group of 'medical insomniacs', clinical advice and treatment are the best and most effective way of proceeding.

But many, perhaps most of those insomniacs who do go to a doctor aren't very happy with the outcome. They don't want to take sleeping pills under any circumstances; or they don't feel that the doctor's advice, however well considered, was of any help.

And anyway, the majority of insomniacs never go to their doctor. They either suffer in silence, or self medicate. And most of the ones who do tell their doctor about their sleep problem only raise it while seeing him or her about other unrelated conditions. As a nation, we are peculiarly hesitant about seeking help for sleeplessness. Perhaps we think that somehow it's an admission of failure, or of weakness.

But perhaps it's just as well that only 1 in every 256 insomniacs asks for medical help. UK doctors dish out 215,000,000 prescriptions for hypnotics per annum, making sleeping pills one of the most popular types of medication. If everyone with insomnia wanted a prescription, it would use up the entire NHS drugs budget!

Reference

CITA (Council for Involuntary Tranquilliser Addiction)
  Cavendish House
  Brighton Road
  Waterloo
  Liverpool
  L22 5NG
  tel: 051-949 0102

CHAPTER 3

Why sleep goes wrong

Insomnia is, if you'll forgive the phrase, a blanket term. There are many different ways of sleeping badly, or inappropriately. The International Classification of Sleep Disorders now lists no fewer than eighty-four conditions associated with some abnormality of sleep. Some of them are vanishingly rare; others are more prevalent. All together, they affect a good third of the population.

As a rule of thumb, women are more likely than men to be affected by insomnia; there are four women with sleeping difficulties for every three men. As a result, women take more sleeping pills, and are more likely to have dependency problems. It is not known why women are more at risk, but there are various theories which may explain the sex difference. Some believe that women are more prone to brood on stressful or unpleasant events than men, who are more likely to externalise their worries. Others think that the higher incidence of insomnia in middle-aged and older women may well be due to broken sleep patterns during child-rearing producing their effects 15–25 years later in life.

What is certain is that the incidence of insomnia increases with age, although it is by no means certain why. It's well known that there is more daytime napping, and more episodes of waking through the night as you get older. This is why the elderly sleeper often complains of not feeling rested in the morning. In addition, older men with prostate problems often have to make three, four or more trips to the loo during the night, which does nothing for the quality of sleep.

13

Some people believe that the circuits in the brain which regulate sleep simply 'wear out' with age. Others believe that the change in sleeping patterns is contributed to by the absence of social pressures, such as the need to fit one's life around a work schedule. A third group of sleep scientists think that reduced physical activity during the day, typical of many elderly subjects, is important in denying core sleep during the night.

TOP TEN SLEEP DISORDERS

Below is a list of the ten most important types of sleep disorder, with an indication as to how common they are, and who they are likely to affect.

1. Nightmares
Nearly half of children aged 3–5 have nightmares on an intermittent or fairly regular basis. Nearly as many adults have infrequent nightmares, and in an unhappy 1 per cent they occur regularly. A sign of stress, and occasionally, difficult sleeping conditions.

Equal 2. Sleep paralysis
That feeling of running in treacle, or a more general inability to move. Worrying, but nothing to be frightened of; about 50 per cent of the population experience occasional episodes. The only cure for sleep paralysis would be to stop sleeping, or at least stop dreaming, but neither of these options is really practical. Better to learn to live with it.

Equal 2. Snoring
Half of over-65s snore, and not a few younger men and women too. Nose clips, tennis balls sewn into the back of the pyjama jacket or even a gentle kick can all help. (See Chapter 5 on snoring.)

3. Sleep enuresis

A third of four-year-old children wet their beds. By age six this has dropped to 10 per cent, and at ten fewer than 5 per cent still have the habit. It can be a sign of unhappiness, and certainly makes the child and parents very unhappy. A sensitive and sympathetic talking to can often help; if not, there is a variety of electronic warning devices which buzz, bleep or whistle to wake the child if they register moisture, which are sometimes effective.

4. Restless legs

Less painful than leg cramps, but just as unbearable. This baffling medical condition affects up to 15 per cent of healthy people, but as many as 30 per cent of patients with rheumatoid arthritis. It can be triggered by iron deficiency, or excessive tea drinking, and can sometimes be treated with iron supplements and by switching to Horlicks or herbal teas. Some people are helped by large doses of vitamin E

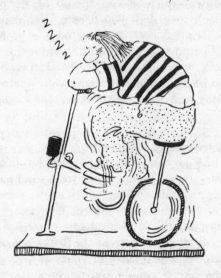

RESTLESS LEGS

15

(about 800 IUs daily), or folic acid, at 5mg one to three times a day.

5. Nocturnal leg cramps
As many as 16 per cent of healthy people get leg cramps, which as any sufferer can tell you are excruciatingly painful. Stretch the limb as much as you can, place the foot in a bucket of hot water and massage as hard as you can tolerate. To make attacks less likely, try Dolomite tablets. Alternatively, some people swear by fish oil. If you decide to try fish oil, eschew bottled oils, which go off too quickly, and try instead a good quality fish oil in capsule form.

6. Sleepwalking
This slightly unnerving condition plagues as many as 15 per cent of people at some time in their lives. It is more common in children than in adults, and often (but not exclusively) associated with the less common night terrors. Sleepwalking children should be gently but firmly steered back to bed. If you dream that you are walking down the High Street wearing only a pyjama top, and wake up to find yourself standing shivering outside Barclay's Bank, you've probably been sleepwalking too. The cure could be as simple as getting your partner to lock the door, hiding the key and making the house as safe as possible.

7. Shift-work-related insomnia
As many as 5 per cent of the population has insomnia related to shift working conditions. Shift work (and particularly the vicious rotating shift system, which keeps workers' circadian rhythms under constant pressure), is a victory for Mammon over human health. Some production processes simply can't shut down overnight – such as the float glass production line at Pilkington's, which runs for years at a time, or strategic institutions like hospitals and power stations. Sleep/wake cycles out of synch with the standard day/night, light/dark

cycle are asking for trouble. There are remedies (see Chapter 13).

8. Night terrors

Reckoned to affect 3 per cent of children, and a few adults. The sufferer experiences extreme but indefinable terror, and is discovered sitting up in bed, screaming. Highly disturbing to parents and partners, and in some ways night terrors are even worse for them. Come the dawn, they'll remember the whole awful episode – but the screamer won't.

9. Obstructive sleep apnoea syndrome (OSAS)

Two per cent of sleepers (but mostly middle-aged and over-weight men) have OSAS. This condition is more alarming to the sleeper's partner than the sleeper himself, as it consists of increasingly laboured breathing, and abrupt cessation of breathing altogether for periods of up to 50 or even 60 seconds at a time. At the end of this time a spasm, a snort and the restoration of snoring will reassure you that he's still in the land of the living, but for anyone with bad OSAS, the long-term prospects are less than rosy. (See Chapter 5 on snoring.)

10. Narcolepsy

An estimated 0.15 per cent of the population suffer from narcolepsy, or sudden and inappropriate sleep. A dangerous disorder, and associated with a ten-fold increase in the rate of road accidents.

CHAPTER 4

Nightmares and night terrors

ROBERT'S STORY

'Funnily enough, I used to get a lot of nightmares as a kid. And it was always the same one. I had scarlet fever when I was eight, and I used to dream I was rocking around in a wooden hut on the sea. The wall would break down and the sea would come flooding in, bringing monsters with it. I would wake screaming, sweating and crying, and for quite a while, I couldn't get to sleep again unless my mother took me into her bed. There, the dreams were of ladies dancing in beautiful dresses!

'Now I'm older, I can see how that four-month disturbed sleep period was largely psychological. I needed a comforter to get real sleep – and that lay with my parents. I recently suffered another spell of nightmares when things were going badly with my business. They would usually take the same pattern, ending with the bailiffs breaking down the door – weirdly, that is not so dissimilar to the hut wall of my childhood and the nasty monsters. I would wake completely sweating and revved up – far too hyped up to get back to sleep. Business is still bad, but what I now try to do is mentally clear the decks before bedtime. Any leftover jobs I would normally put off to the next day, I try and deal with. I then try to "switch off" with some mindless TV or a chapter of a book, so that I don't take my problems to bed. All I can say is that the nightmares have stopped, thank goodness!'

WHAT IS A NIGHTMARE?

A nightmare is basically just a bad dream, and like other dreams occurs when the brain is in REM or the rapid eye movement phase of sleep. They can be extremely complex, colourful and bizarre; or they can be relatively empty, and yet still leave you feeling overwhelmed by some sort of threat. In either case, a nightmare can frighten you awake with a pounding heart, covered in sweat, and feeling generally shaken and apprehensive.

They do not seem to be specifically linked to eating any kinds of foods (although the worst nightmare I can remember, which involved an elephant sitting on my chest, was triggered by indigestion caused by eating a late-night dinner which consisted mostly of cheese); but they do seem to occur

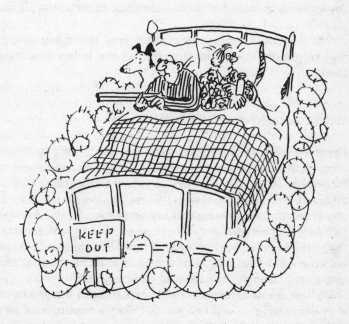

19

more often in individuals who are unwell, or under severe stress. They can be a signal to slow down, and a few of these bad dreams may even give you clues about what exactly is going wrong in your life that is causing the stress.

Chronic nightmares like Robert's story, and particularly those which centre around recurrent themes, are probably telling you something else. In this situation, the recurring elements are more likely to indicate some repressed unpleasant emotion or experience, which for some reason you have been unable to deal with. So you put it out of your mind. But even if you don't think of it during the day, the incident has lodged somewhere in the brain and, when your conscious defences are down, it crops up night after night in symbolised form. It is important to confront these nightmares, either on your own or preferably with someone sympathetic, such as a counsellor or other therapist, in order to unravel the symbolism and defuse the tensions causing the nightmare.

Nightmares are commonest in children, and in adults with post-traumatic stress disorder, but no one is immune from them.

WHAT ARE NIGHT TERRORS?

Night terrors, on the other hand, are quite different, and occur almost exclusively in children. They are not necessarily associated with REM sleep, but occur early at night, soon after entering the deep stage of sleep. The dream imagery, if any is recalled, often seems scanty and insignificant. And yet the child will be sitting up in bed, eyes staring, and screaming at the top of his or her lungs. The oddest thing is that the sufferer will have little, if any, memory of the event in the morning, although the parent(s) certainly will.

Waking up hearing your child screaming in terror can be very distressing, so what do you do? Simple reassurance isn't always effective, but it's the only thing worth trying. Try taking the child gently in your arms, and if this doesn't make matters worse try rocking him or her very gently. Reassure him or her that you're there, and that everything is all right, nothing has happened. Eventually the child will calm down, and fall asleep as if nothing untoward had occurred.

It's not know what causes night terrors, but they do run in families, so there may be a genetic susceptibility; and they seem to occur more frequently in children under severe stress. They may, for example, be a symptom of a child suffering from bullying, or whose parents are going through a particularly bad time.

The child who experiences night terrors may also be a sleepwalker, as the two conditions often go together. If there is a sleepwalking child in your family, take basic precautions. Don't leave the Ming where he or she could stumble into it, and don't leave trailing wires, cables or other obstacles on the ground where they are likely to walk. Make sure, also, that there are no open windows within easy reach. Even so, many sleepwalkers harm themselves during their midnight ramblings, so if you should see one, steer him or her gently back into bed. You almost certainly won't wake the sleepwalker, and even if you do it won't do any harm. As with the night terrors, calm and gentle reassurance is the best approach.

CHAPTER 5

Snoring

It's amazing how loudly some people can snore, but if you live with a snorer, you probably think he or she has the loudest snore in the world – especially if it's keeping you awake at night. In fact, the loudest snore known to man, as recorded in the *Guinness Book of Records*, was emitted by Canadian Mark Hubbard. At his peak, he hit a stunning 90 decibels – 10 decibels louder than the local noise limits for traffic! And the case of an elderly woman from Leeds was reported recently in the newspapers when local magistrates decided her snoring was loud enough to be in contravention of the Control of Pollution (Noise) Act.

It's even more amazing when you realise that these people, and others like them, are regularly deafening their partners, terrorising small animals and young children, rattling the windows and even waking the neighbours – but incredibly they can do all this without waking themselves.

Snoring is caused by the soft palate, at the back of the roof of the mouth, vibrating during inhalation like a sail flapping in the wind. It seems to be age-related, as below the age of thirty-five or so snorers are in a minority. One in five men, and a mere one in twenty women regularly snore. But by the time you're ready to collect your pension, the snorers have taken over. Two thirds of men, and nearly half the women in this age group are confirmed snorers.

Being overweight is a predisposing factor; a collar size of 17 or over practically guarantees snoring. Surprisingly, the tongue is one of the first parts of the body to get fat, and as this happens it reduces the size of the oropharyngeal lumen (or airway) through which air passes, making snoring more likely. Excess alcohol consumption also tends to make the problem worse. And as we are, as a nation, running ever more to fat, the problem of snoring is getting steadily more common.

Snoring is no joke for the unfortunate people whose partners (mostly, but not exclusively male) snore. It can drive them into a wild rage, or the divorce courts, and sometimes even further – in a few documented cases, victims of chronic snoring have resorted to murder to finally achieve an undisturbed night's sleep. And it is no joke for the snorer either. Researchers in sleep labs have found that a significant number of snorers suffer from sleep apnoea, or sleep breathlessness. It is particularly prevalent in overweight and obese people, and can be quite frightening to watch.

The soft tissues at the back of the throat relax, fall in on one another and finally close, stopping all respiration. The sleeper typically makes a few false starts, and movements, but breathing may not resume for as much as a minute. As levels of oxygen in the blood fall, the brain detects that something is wrong, and sends increasingly urgent messages to the breathing muscles to start working. The sleeper takes a few violent, gasping breaths and then settles back into the more regular snoring. Through the night he (or she) alternates between the two types of breathing, tossing and turning restlessly but never completely waking.

The near awakenings are so brief that the subject is rarely aware of them, but they may occur many hundreds of times a night, disrupting core sleep and ensuring that the sleeper spends more time in the less restorative and lighter Stage 1 and 2 sleep. The next morning the victim typically feels hung over, with headaches and fatigue, drowsiness and mental dulling which last through the day.

If you notice that your partner suffers from this particular type of snoring then you should seriously consider a trip to the doctor, because sleep apnoea has been linked to an increased risk of heart attack. The periods of low oxygen, and the resulting release into the blood of floods of adrenalin, speed up the heartbeat and make it more unstable. If there is any underlying cardiac problem, this can be enough to trigger a heart attack or arrythmia, which can be fatal. The increase in blood pressure probably explains why sleep apnoea is also linked with a greater than normal risk of a stroke; although the fact that most apnoeac snorers are overweight is also a contributory factor.

A reduction in intelligence has also been reported in some sleep apnoeacs, and here the cause is thought to be the prolonged periods of oxygen starvation. The brain is highly sensitive to low oxygen concentrations, and repeated hours of low oxygen may be sufficient to cause minimal brain damage. Personality changes have also been noted; although whether these were due to brain damage, or simply a reflection of chronic fatigue, has never been proven. Whatever the cause, people who suffer from sleep apnoea often experience marital friction and breakdown, and difficulties at work.

Strange noises aside, sleep apnoea is no laughing matter. If you or your partner suffer from sleep apnoea, then it is advisable to seek medical help. Weight loss may be enough, and cutting down on alcohol intake will also help. Sleeping pills only make the problem worse, and must be avoided. There may be other problems, such as nasal conditions which need attention, or other underlying illnesses which could be treated.

HOW TO STOP SNORING

Yes, it sounds a lot like the revenge of the restless, but the tried and trusted favourite is sewing a tennis ball or even half a cricket ball into the back of the pyjamas, so that the sleeper will tend to stay off his or her back; once on their side, the airways are much less prone to blocking. A second device is the vibration sensor, worn on the wrist, which detects when the wearer has gone into snoring mode. It then starts to buzz in a very irritating way, and is supposed to wake the wearer sufficiently to make him roll over, and stop snoring.

There are a few treatments which act directly on the spot. The first, which is by far the cheapest and safest, and is more suitable for the non-apnoeac snorer, involves a small plastic device which clips to the nose, and holds the nostrils wide open so as to make nose breathing easier. This helps some snorers, but the sight is irresistibly comic and can provoke fits of raucous laughter in the non-snorer, which are invariably counter-productive.

In more serious cases a mask is worn over the nose and mouth, to deliver air at a slightly higher pressure than normal. It keeps the airways open; it starts working the moment you put it on, and helps the vast majority of patients – over 99 per cent, according to some estimates. Patients report dramatic improvements in their well-being, saying that they feel more rested in the morning and suffer less daytime sleepiness. But you have to wear the mask every night, which some people don't like. It might work reasonably well in the context of an established relationship, but how would you feel about the mask if, for example, you were only just beginning to get to know your sleeping partner?

If all else fails, and for the avowedly self-conscious, there is an anti-snoring operation. This is a relatively minor surgical procedure, which is done on a day-patient basis, but it is obviously the last resort. The surgeon cauterises the soft palate, creating scar tissue, which makes it more rigid and less likely to flap, or fold inwards and block the airways. The operation is called uvulopalatopharyngoplasty. Even at eleven syllables, it doesn't always work, but in some patients it does produce improvement. Other procedures are being developed, but are, at the time of writing, even more experimental.

When sleep apnoea occurs in schoolchildren, the daytime 'hangover' effect can damage their scholastic progress. In these cases, the cause of the apnoea is often enlarged tonsils, and sometimes adenoids, and surgery is indicated.

The last, and in some ways oddest, group of sleep apnoeacs are body builders. The anabolic steroids that so many of them take can cause a build-up of tissue in the neck and throat which obstructs the airways – so the next time you watch the well-known Hollywood musclemen going through their paces on screen, stop a moment to reflect on what they sound like when they sleep. It's a sobering prospect. And if any would-be body builder is reading this book, avoid nandrolone, which seems to be particularly prone to causing this problem.

CHAPTER 6

Categories of insomnia – which one are you?

There are many different factors which can bring on insomnia. The recent Royal Society of Medicine Round Table series No 28 lists over twenty. Working medics, however, use a handy short list called the '5 Ps', which covers most of the common causes of insomnia. The 5 Ps are as follows:

1. Physical
2. Physiological
3. Pharmacological
4. Psychological
5. Psychiatric

1. PHYSICAL

This category includes sleep-denying illnesses such as heart disease, asthma, gastric reflux and other indigestion problems. Any other physical condition which causes chronic pain is likely to have the same effect, and tinnitus (ringing in the ears) and prostate problems are also high on the list. And don't forget myoclonus akathisia (medicalese for sudden movements of the limbs, which can startle you awake) and leg cramps.

2. PHYSIOLOGICAL

Under Physiological, file: late-night eating, which boosts the metabolism. Late-night exercise, if too strenuous, will also keep you awake; in fact, anything that causes too much excitement and arousal will have the same effect, whether it's anger, or the nervous thrills of a good horror movie.

3. PHARMACOLOGICAL

Caffeine, alcohol, nicotine, and various medically prescribed drugs such as beta blockers (anti-hypertensives) and some anti-depressants, are all capable of ruining a good night's sleep. Users of illegal drugs such as cocaine, amphetamines and crack will also experience severe sleeping difficulties.

4. PSYCHOLOGICAL

Bereavement, loss of or change of employment, and other major life events often trigger sleeping difficulties. Any cause of stress or tension, whether chronic or acute, will cause problems. Then there's sleep neurosis, an abnormal concern about not sleeping, a slightly bizarre but surprisingly common syndrome where fear of the problem of insomnia actually brings it about; post-traumatic stress disorder, which may affect the survivors of accidents and disasters; and, sadly, those with a history of childhood abuse, who learned early on to associate the bedroom with pain, danger, and threat, are often sufferers.

This last category is a special form of insomnia which is best described as conditioned insomnia; and there are many other less dramatic examples of this, where sleeping difficulties can be traced back to childhood events and habits. For example, in can occur in children who were sent to bed early for being naughty, a form of punishment that is perhaps less popular than it used to be. Those children grow into adults who may still, at a subconscious level, associate the bedroom and going to bed with anger, frustration and punishment.

Parents who send their children to bed purely to get them out of the way, leaving them lying awake, bored and resentful, could be laying the foundations of a habit of sleeplessness that could well come back to haunt the children in adulthood. Negative feelings about self and the bedroom environment can be worsened if the child overhears the parent or parents fighting, perhaps over the child, or alternatively having a good time somewhere else in the house. The bedroom becomes tainted with feelings of unhappiness, or being left out. Later in life, going to bed can unlock those memories, allowing feelings of insecurity and unease to well up to the surface. Mixed in with current worries and stresses, they create a mindset which is hardly conducive to getting a good night's sleep.

5. PSYCHIATRIC

Several of the major psychiatric illnesses are associated with sleeping problems, but the most common conditions are the anxiety states, depressive illness and mania.

PMORE

The above list is by no means complete. A sixth category of common causes of insomnia is referred to, somewhat bafflingly, as 'sleep hygiene'. This refers to such insomnia-inducing habits as taking too many daytime naps. It also covers the bedroom milieu, affecting such issues as: how comfortable is the bed? Is the bedroom at the right temperature? (An excessively hot or cold bedroom makes it difficult to sleep well.) Is there enough room in the bed? Do your feet hang out over the end? How many adults, children or animals do you share it with? etc.

That hardy urban perennial, noise, comes in here – neighbours' parties, music from the flat upstairs, or traffic are the bane of many a city-dwelling insomniac's life – so how peaceful is your bedroom, and are noise levels important to you? (Some people seem to require almost complete quiet to sleep well, while others will plug themselves into a Walkman to get their night's repose.) And, critically for many, does your partner snore?

No idle question, this, because it leads naturally to our next problem area, namely, the seventh category of sleep disorders which are not strictly speaking insomnia, but which are also associated with disturbed sleep. The most common of these is snoring, and especially sleep apnoea (see Chapter 5 on snoring). Alongside snoring in this catch-all category of sleep disturbances are sleepwalking, night terrors, enuresis (bed-wetting), and bruxism (teeth-grinding, which, like snoring, is more likely to wake the sleeper's partner or parent(s) than the sleeper).

Finally, there are several conditions associated with feelings of tiredness, fatigue and lack of energy, which are not actually sleep disorders, even though patients will often complain of very similar symptoms. The three most commonly diagnosed are ME (myalgic encephalitis, which was once known as 'Yuppie flu'); CFS (Chronic Fatigue Syndrome); and TATT, yet another medical acronym which stands for Tired All The Time (see Chapter 7). And in addition to the above, sub-clinical deficiencies of certain nutrients can also leave the sufferer feeling tired and lethargic.

CHAPTER 7

Tired all the time

Measuring energy levels is difficult, but we all know the difference between feeling vital and alive, and feeling tired and lethargic. And although illness or late nights can leave you drained, the main factor in determining whether you feel energetic or comatose is what you eat.

We're eating more processed foods than ever before, which are often high in calories but low in nutrition. As a result, more of us risk becoming deficient in certain key nutrients, which can cause low energy. Dieters are particularly vulnerable, not only because calorie restriction slows down the metabolism, but also because many diets are nutritionally poor.

There is in addition a possible link between tiredness and low blood pressure. The Germans have long been convinced that there is a link between fatigue and low blood pressure – usually more common in women than men – yet in Britain, you are usually congratulated if your blood pressure is low. The most commonly prescribed drug in Germany for this condition is Digoxin, which is used in tiny amounts to boost the pressure.

As many as one in three women may be suffering from iron-deficiency anaemia. Symptoms include fatigue and pallor – particularly inside the eyelid. If this describes you, your doctor may recommend an iron supplement. Chromium deficiency is thought to be very common too. The symptoms include a craving for sweet foods, weight gain, and loss of energy – all of which can be helped with chromium supplements.

These conditions are relatively clearly defined, and

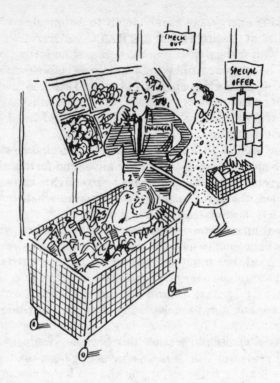

TIRED ALL THE TIME

respond well to specific nutritional therapy. Other conditions, such as TATT (Tired All The Time), ME (Myalgic encephalitis) and CFS (Chronic Fatigue Syndrome) are less easy to categorise and there is a great deal of controversy among the medical profession as to what they are, or indeed, if they are different conditions at all.

TATT

TATT is a somewhat mysterious ailment which is intermittently popular. People with TATT complain of being tired and lacking energy, but rarely admit to feeling sleepy. And that is what distinguishes the TATT sufferer from the patient with a sleep disturbance, because the latter do feel sleepy. The apnoeac patient for example will often doze off in the daytime, when watching TV or when sitting in the bus, the train or the passenger seat of the car – and sometimes even at the wheel. TATT patients on the other hand don't tend to sleep during the day.

So how is TATT treated? It depends very much on the doctor. Some prescribe sleeping pills, although there is a growing consensus that these don't help, and can often make the problem of lethargy and low energy worse. Other doctors believe that in some cases TATT, like insomnia, may have a psychiatric origin, and tend to look for an underlying illness such as depression, which could be specifically treated. But you may find that many doctors – perhaps your own GP – take a more robust view, and maintain that the best treatment for TATT is TOTT (Turn Off The Television), which is really a variant on the much older medical strategy of PYSU (Pull Your Socks Up). Patients are advised in addition to take more exercise and get to bed earlier.

LOUISE'S STORY

'Ever since I was a child, I can remember feeling tired all the time – what an appropriate name for it! Now I'm an adult, and I've done something positive about my TATT, I can see that that is not normal in a child. I'm normal weight for my height, I don't get colds and hardly suffer from flu; I thought I was eating properly – yet all my waking thoughts seemed to centre on how exhausted I felt. I actually didn't get a very positive response from my GP, so on the advice of a friend, I went to a homeopath. It was a really in-depth consultation. She asked hundreds of questions and examined my body. She worked out that I had an iron deficiency and thought also that glandular fever, which I got as a teenager, was still lurking in my system. She prescribed various medicines and told me to cut down on caffeine and sugar and drink plenty of water. I was also told to eat little and often so that I wouldn't get those dips of energy during the day. I also joined a gym – very unlike me – and now do a gentle exercise routine each day. The result three months later is that I wake up naturally early each morning, which is a definite first for me, and I can seem to keep going throughout the day that much longer. I wish I had done something about it in my twenties!

ME

And then there is ME, subject of much debate, which is also known as Persistent Virus Disease. Some doctors think that TATT and ME are indistinguishable, and that they are both fancy names for malingering, but there is some evidence that ME may have an organic cause. Some scientists have found evidence for a persistent viral infection in parts of the central nervous system (hence ME's alternative title). As a result, ME is now recognised by the World Health Organisation as a neurological disorder, and it does seem that the estimated 150,000 British ME sufferers form a quite distinct group. Symptoms of severe exercise intolerance and extreme alcohol sensitivity should alert doctors to a possible ME diagnosis. The best treatment is thought to be traditional bed rest; exercise can actually make ME worse. For further information write to ME Action.

CFS

Chronic Fatigue Syndrome (CFS) is considered to be a sequel to glandular fever and some other viral infections. In distinct contrast to ME, CFS is best treated with progressive exercise routines to gradually build up strength and energy levels. It is claimed that CFS can also be brought on by psychiatric conditions such as depression and anxiety or panic disorders, although in these cases a diagnosis of TATT might equally well be made; and here, treatment should be aimed at the underlying psychiatric illness.

Self Help

1. Consider taking a vitamin supplement, but see a nutritionalist for the best advice.
2. If you are anaemic, don't drink tea or coffee during meals. They inhibit the absorption of iron by between 40 per cent and 60 per cent. Take an iron supplement and help it along by eating plenty of iron-rich foods like green leafy vegetables, pulses, liver and egg yolks. Taking 500mg of vitamin C will also help.
3. If fatigue is chronic, as in Chronic Fatigue Syndrome, and not due to stress, anaemia or any of the other common factors, investigate food sensitivities.
4.. Clean up your dietary act – cut down on stimulants, and don't rely on sugar for a quick energy fix.
5. Tackle the problem with an alternative therapy: try aromatherapy oils, especially neroli, lavender or ylang-ylang (see later chapters).

Reference

ME Action
  PO Box 1302
  Wells
  BA5 2WE

Get Up and Go! by Anne Woodham (Headline, £5.99)

CHAPTER 8

Sleep and health

Stage 3 and 4 sleep are often referred to collectively as core sleep, and are thought to be essential for our physical well-being. Sleep deprivation experiments have shown that after people have been kept awake for several days, they don't need to catch up on all the sleep that they missed – but they do, very rapidly, recover all the lost core sleep.

The importance of core sleep was also demonstrated in experiments where volunteers slept for only a half-hour every 4 hours, for weeks at a time, without adverse effects on their health or work performance. Their total sleep time was only 2 to 3 hours a day – but it was nearly all core sleep.

What's more, people who naturally do not sleep for very long get as much core sleep as anyone; it's the Stage 1 and 2 sleep they cut down on. It seems possible that people can train themselves, either deliberately or as the result of social pressures, to do without Stage 1 and 2 sleep; some scientists believe that this is little more than 'filler', just a way of conserving energy in the dark hours between dusk and dawn.

So what's so special about core sleep? Well, one aspect of core sleep is that it triggers the release, from the pituitary gland located just below the brain, of Growth Hormone (GH). GH is responsible for the growth and repair of muscle, bone, gut, spleen and many other tissues.

The sleep-related release of Growth Hormone explains why rates of tissue repair are highest during sleep. In children and adolescents, the rate of bone growth increases at night for just this reason, which suggests that the old idea that late nights stunt growth may well have something in it.

Interestingly enough, treatment of short stature with GH is more effective if it is given at night, rather than during the day.

When the need for growth is greatest (such as during pregnancy, adolescence, or the building up of patients recovering from anorexia), the duration of sleep and slow-wave sleep, and the amount of GH released, all increase. A similar response occurs when daily energy expenditure is raised, either through increased exercise, or in some medical conditions such as hyperthyroidism. But when we use less energy, the amount of slow-wave sleep, and GH release, is reduced. (See Chapter 17 on sleep and exercise.)

When we say that the rate of tissue growth and repair is greatest at night, what this means is that this is the time when our body cells are most active, and when they are most actively dividing (which they must do in order to multiply). This is why lack of sleep shows up first in the skin. The skin cells are constantly being replaced, which keeps the skin clean and healthy, and a large part of the renewal takes place at night, during slow-wave sleep. If we don't get enough of this restorative sleep, the rate of skin cell replacement slows down, and our skin loses its clarity and bloom.

The fact that slow-wave sleep is so intimately linked with growth and repair solves several medical puzzles. It explains, for example, why patients with medical conditions that disrupt sleep complain that the effects of their condition on their quality of life are worse than those whose sleep is not disturbed. It also explains why patients with severe chronic insomnia and those who take drugs, including sleeping pills, which disrupt their normal sleep patterns, have slightly shorter life spans.

This last idea, that insomnia can be life-shortening, is what one might expect, in an intuitive sort of way. Anything which damages or blocks our normal behavioural patterns could well have some sort of damaging effect. But where is the hard evidence?

The first clues come from a survey of 9,000 UK adults

which found that the lucky group who slept a normal amount (that is, between 6$\frac{1}{2}$ and 8$\frac{1}{2}$ hours), suffered from fewer illnesses. Hot on its heels came the report of an American Cancer Society study of over a million volunteers, who were enrolled into the study and then followed up for six years. The scientists found an unexpected increase in the death rate in people with chronic sleeping problems who, as a consequence, often took sleeping pills.

Unfairly, women come off worse. Sleeping problems appear to increase the death rate by half in women, and by a quarter in men, whose sleep is either two hours shorter *or longer* than the norm. In fact, several more large studies have now shown that insomnia is as powerful a predictor of early death as obesity.

Most of the popular books on insomnia omit this uncomfortable fact, either because the authors were unaware of the data, or possibly because they didn't want to worry their readers. And they have a point, because a fair number of people worry so much about not getting to sleep that their worry keeps them, paradoxically, awake. The last thing anyone wants to do is to add to insomniacs' worries, and risk making their sleep disorder worse.

However, I strongly believe that what you don't know can still hurt you – and is in fact more likely to hurt you than information that you can take on board, and deal with. So don't panic, because in this book you will find collections of remedies that will help your sleeping problems and tilt the odds back in your favour.

CHAPTER 9

Duration of insomnia: is this you?

We've looked at some of the many causes of sleeping problems, and some of the systems of classification of the different types of insomnia. Now, to confirm your suspicions about the slight woolliness of this area of study, here's another formula the medics use when deciding on what course of treatment they should prescribe. It is based not on the cause, but the duration of the insomnia, and according to this system insomnia is divided into three types:

1. TRANSIENT (several days): caused by such factors as acute stress, environmental factors and jet lag. Treatment (in order of preference): sleeping pills, advice, counselling.
2. SHORT TERM (up to three weeks): caused by family problems, emotional distress, illness, bereavement, shift work. Preferred treatment: counselling, advice, sleeping pills.
3. CHRONIC (months to years): caused by chronic conditions such as asthma, arthritis, dementia. Preferred treatment: treating the underlying medical condition, counselling, sleeping pills.

The main difference in treatment options is that as the insomnia progresses from acute to chronic, sleeping pills become less popular. Most doctors would agree that transient and short-term insomnia responds better to sleeping pills or hypnotics, and prefer not to use them for chronic insomnia. This is not necessarily because they do not work, although some long-term patients do eventually become resistant to them, but if the insomnia is long term, then the hypnotics may also need to be given on a long-term basis – and the risk of dependency becomes more substantial.

Even when prescribing sleeping pills for short-term use, doctors are nowadays very careful. They will give you pills for a few days only, because they want to avoid a slide into long-term use. After bereavement, for example, they are unlikely to prescribe more than four or five days' worth, to avoid impairing the normal and healthy compensatory coping reactions to stress. If sleeping problems persist, they will then generally recommend counselling or other non-drug therapy if needed.

INSOMNIA SELF CHECK

If you can identify your type of insomnia, and pinpoint the main cause or causes of the sleep disturbance, then congratulations! You've already gone a considerable way towards solving the problem. The following check-list identifies the five most common types of insomnia, and lists their main causes.

Type A: Takes far too long to get to sleep
This type of insomnia is most common in the under-30s, and in women.

Causes include:
★ Conditioned insomnia (problems deriving from childhood)
★ Emotional stress of any origin, whether relating to past or future events
★ Dwelling on unsolved problems
★ Obsessional thoughts (e.g. is my partner unfaithful?)
★ Dietary factors (such as eating too late, or drinking coffee in bed)

★ Digestive problems
★ Medical conditions, including any which cause severe or sustained pain
★ Inactive lifestyle
★ Daytime napping
★ Going to bed too early – i.e. trying to get more sleep than you actually need
★ Disturbed body clocks, caused by jet lag or shift work
★ Environmental factors, such as noisy neighbours or street life
★ Bad sleep hygiene (such as an unsuitable bed or bedroom)

Type B: Wakes during the night

This type of insomnia is more common in elderly people. Many of the factors which can trigger type A insomnia can give rise to type B as well, but in addition there are a number of factors which give rise solely to type B.

Causes include:
★ Intense anger and irritability
★ Heavy alcohol consumption
★ Withdrawal symptoms from alcohol, sleeping pills or other drugs
★ Nightmares – and if these are frequent, fear of nightmares (Some insomniacs learn to wake before dreaming begins.)
★ Anorexia (The insomnia stops once normal eating is resumed.)
★ Menopause (HRT treats the night sweats, which are quite common, and usually restores healthy, pre-menopausal sleep patterns.)

Type C: Wakes too early

Many of the factors which trigger types A and B insomnia can give rise to type C as well, but in addition there are several factors which predispose solely to type C.

Causes include:
★ Severe depression
★ Alcoholism

Type D: Getting enough sleep but still feeling tired
This is a rogue category.

Causes include:
★ Sleep apnoea
★ Depression
★ Other causes of low energy
★ Pseudo-insomnia (see below)

Pseudo-insomnia
This is one of the most baffling sleep disorders of all. People with pseudo-insomnia fall asleep readily enough, and get the right amount of sleep, but complain in the morning that they haven't slept – and in a funny way, they're telling the truth. Recent research in sleep labs has revealed that in a small minority of people, previously categorised as malingerers or hypochondriacs, there is a deficiency of deep or core sleep. Their brains are not very good at manufacturing or producing this kind of sleep, so they spend the night in Stages 1 and 2 sleep and maintain a degree of awareness of their surroundings which deeper sleepers do not have. This means that they are aware of moving position in the bed during the night, and hear the chimes of the local clock, even though they are technically asleep. Their brain traces suggest that some pseudo-insomniacs spend the night thinking about something; in some cases, dreaming that they are awake.

Type E: Not getting enough sleep, but not feeling tired

Cause:
★ Sleep Neurosis

This strange condition describes the self-professed insomniac, who is in fact getting as much sleep as he or she needs. Sleep lab studies show that in some cases, people who complain of an inability to get to sleep are actually falling asleep quite normally, but overestimate the time they spend lying awake simply because they're worried about not being able to fall asleep!

Almost by definition, sleep neurosis is difficult to self diagnose. If you don't have access to a sleep lab, an accurate diagnosis is probably best made by a partner – but unfortunately sufferers are notoriously reluctant to accept a partner's word for it. Here is an alternative and less disputatious approach to self diagnosis. Put a clock by the bed, where it can easily be seen. Leave a notepad and pencil on the bedside table, and every 30 minutes, note down the time in your sleep log. In the morning, score the number of entries in the log. Do this for 10 to 14 days; and if you find that you're mostly scoring ones with a few twos, your insomnia is more apparent than real.

The message for this kind of insomniac is basically: don't worry, be happy. You are getting more sleep than you think, and probably as much as you need. And if the sleep log reveals a true insomniac? Well, as long as you're getting some sleep, managing to relax and eating a good diet, your sleeping problem isn't going to do you much harm in the short term, providing you manage to stay awake at the wheel. So try to relax, even if you are lying awake in bed; enjoy feeling cosy and warm, and not having to do anything, because your attitude towards sleep will influence the quality of the sleep you do get.

Remember Sarah's story in Chapter 2? Sarah found that a more positive attitude to sleep really helped her to relax and on many occasions, actually to sleep. When Sarah concentrated on her sleeplessness, it would set off a chain of worrying where all the problems in her life came to the fore:

'I'm sure it had to do with being sent to bed as a punishment when I was little. I'd lie in bed fretting about what I had done wrong, then as an adult, I was repeating those patterns. Bed obviously represented a place of unhappiness for me. I have to force myself to think positive thoughts, but it really works. I run through the day, thinking of all the good things I've achieved. I remember good experiences, and I concentrate on sensations, like the warmth of the bed, the coolness of the pillow. I then try and imagine an enveloping blanket of black velvet and, closing my eyes, I concentrate on that. When I do this, I can actually feel my muscles relax and my mind too!'

CHAPTER 10

Special groups

CHILDREN

Let's face it – babies are true individuals when it comes to sleep patterns, and those under nine months or so who still need a night feed are going to wake up, and often cry, no matter what you do. But after nine months, a baby who consistently cries at night and has sleeping difficulties is actually telling you something quite different.

Older children with sleeping problems are usually children who haven't yet learned to sleep alone, or who have an anxiety problem. Fear of the dark, anxiety about school, or separation from parents, or lack of a fixed routine before sleeping can all cause difficulties. A sleep diary kept by the parents for a few days should show up any pattern, and a simple remedy such as a night light or an intercom can help. (These are great for helping the child to feel in touch with

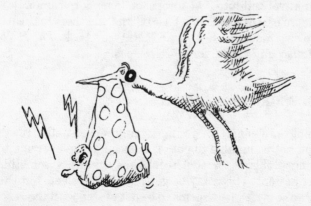

the parents, but be warned – it's all too easy to forget the intercom, and say something that the child shouldn't be hearing! The best models have a toggle switch, and are only live when you specifically want them to be.) Last but not least, develop a simple bedtime routine; a wash, into pyjamas, a story and then bed – and no late-night adult TV!

Some parents let their child cry itself to sleep, but personally I prefer the well-worn 5 minute method. Although a purist might say it's a slightly dishonest approach, it works pretty well and is easy on all parties. You tell the child to lie with eyes lightly closed, waiting to fall asleep, but not to fall asleep just yet because Mum or Dad will be back to see everything's all right in 5 minutes, and not before. Go back when the 5 minutes are up, reassure and comfort the child if necessary, and leave the room before he/she falls asleep – because you'll be back in another 5 minutes. Repeat, until the child falls asleep on his or her own. After four or five nights, increase the interval to 10 minutes; and then, in another week or so when the 10 minute routine is working, go on to 15 minutes – and so on. In a short time, most children are falling asleep after the first (and last) visit.

You may also like to try some natural remedies to help a child to sleep. For children, camomile, limeflower or catnip tea, made enticing with some honey, will prove relaxing. Alternatively, dilute two drops of lavender, camomile or geranium essential oils in a base oil and add them to the bath or use as a massage. See Anne McIntyre's book, *The Herbal for Mother and Child*, for more recipes.

ADOLESCENTS

Sleeping problems in younger children usually revolve around not being able to get off to sleep in the evening, but sleeping problems in adolescents may indicate something quite different. They may be getting enough sleep, but their sleep/wake cycle often seems to be out of step with the rest of the world, they go to bed in the early hours and they don't rise before midday. This can be infuriating, but isn't in itself a sign of anything more serious than that old but difficult chestnut – the rebellious teenager.

Displaced sleep/wake cycles can most effectively be restored to normal by putting bedtime back, *not* forward, by about two hours each night. If your beautiful child has developed the habit of going to bed at 1.00 a.m., then the next night he or she should stay up until 3.00 a.m. The day after that bedtime is at 5.00 a.m. then 7.00 a.m., and so on for a week or so until bedtime is more or less back in synch with the rest of the family. This method seems very unlikely but is in fact a lot easier than trying to switch the errant offspring to normal in one go, which just doesn't work, and guarantees sleepless nights and loss of goodwill all round.

Anti-social sleep/wake patterns are inconvenient, but not terribly serious. If, on the other hand, your young son or daughter is actually sleeping less, then other explanations must be looked for. There could be an emotional problem. Extreme dieting and anorexia are well-known sleep inhibitors; and substance abuse, including alcohol and street drugs, could be another possible candidate. In all these cases talking and counselling are essential, and other specialist help may well be needed. Counsellors are trained to get to the root cause of a problem and they offer supportive help, whatever the age of the sufferer. Plenty specialise in adolescent problems; they know how to talk to this age group in a sympathetic way, and with their help you will be able to identify whether or not anorexia or substance abuse is a problem. Convincing your teenager that they need to talk to someone may be difficult and, here, recommendations from friends will help. If a child known to the family has seen a counsellor, it will be much easier to broach the subject with your own child. Once they agree, you are half way there – most kids positively welcome talking about their problems to an independent party; the sheer luxury of having that time to themselves, without interference from you, could well become habit-forming! But more on counselling in Chapter 11.

If, however, your teenagers are going to sleep as normal, but waking up in the night, then you should check to see whether they are suffering from breathing problems. Nocturnal asthma is becoming more common, and obstructive sleep apnoea caused by enlarged tonsils or adenoids is also a possible cause. (The remedy is anti-asthma treatment, and tonsillectomy and adenoidectomy respectively.)

THE ELDERLY

If you've got a parent or grandparent living with you, or an elderly relative, then you will be all too aware that elderly people are particularly prone to insomnia. They have more reasons to have sleep problems: chronic pain, bereavement and loneliness are all more likely to occur in this age group. In addition, the elderly are more sensitive to caffeine; and finally, there is some evidence that the biological clock which regulates our physiological rhythms, like every other part of the body, begins to run down. It works less well, doesn't drive the sleep/wake cycle as efficiently, and becomes less able to sustain periods of either long sleep or wakefulness. As a result, many elderly people nap during the day or doze in the evenings – and this is a recipe for poor nocturnal sleep.

Unreasonable expectations can cause problems too, because if you go to bed unrealistically early, you'll certainly have problems falling asleep. A simple change in bedtime can help here. Inactivity is a strong predisposing factor – the physically and mentally alert tend to be less afflicted with sleeping problems, so anything that encourages more physical and mental activity will tend to improve sleep quality.

Most elderly people crave company and fear boredom. Britain lags far behind Europe in terms of involving elderly relatives in the day-to-day running of family life. If your relative is fairly fit, then encourage him or her to read bedtime stories to the children. They could also be given an easy household chore like light dusting or washing up the cocoa mugs. If they are not so fit and like crosswords, puzzles or games, try and set some time aside to join in. A gentle accompanied walk during the evening will help with relaxation – perhaps a visit from a family friend, or a game of cards, bingo or bridge? The main point is that variety of life and some physical activity are essential to this age group. Stimulation aids relaxation which aids sleep. Without stimulation, you get listlessness, lethargy and disturbed sleep – however old or young you are!

Reference

The Herbal for Mother and Child by Anne McIntyre (Element, £9.99)

CHAPTER 11

An insomniac's progress through the medical system

1. Step 1 – the GP
2. Step 2 – counselling
3. Step 3 – the sleep lab

STEP 1 – THE GP

The insomniac's first encounter with the medical system is usually the GP, who is responsible for diagnosing and treating you, and, if necessary, referring you to a specialist. Here's how a GP might view your problem, and some suggestions about points you can usefully raise during the consultation to get your message across.

Start off on the right foot – and remember that a meeting between you and your doctor is a meeting of experts; your doctor has medical skills and training, but you are the expert on your symptoms, and the effect they are having on your life. And this is important, because there are many different types of sleep problem, and many different ways of experiencing them. A good night's sleep can be hard to define – unlike, say, a broken leg. One person's idea of a good night's repose might seem like an endlessly sleepless night to someone else; a lack of sleep may be more of a disaster to one person than another.

This means that it's important to tell the GP as much about the nature of your sleeping problem and how it affects your well-being as possible. We've already seen how many

50

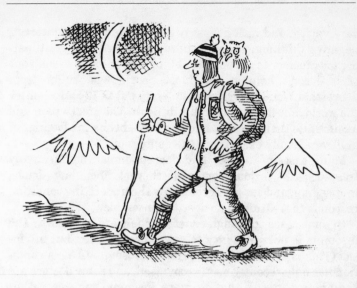

AN INSOMNIAC'S PROGRESS

different kinds of sleep disturbances there are; simply announcing that you are an insomniac won't help very much, and can even be counter-productive, because you're giving the doctor a diagnosis rather than the symptoms. Some GPs are put off by patients who come to them with a ready-made diagnosis – and to be fair on the doctor, he or she does need to know whether there were any events, signs or symptoms which appeared before the sleep problem. They can then consider possible causes, rather than just the end result of the insomnia itself.

Sometimes people are only too aware of the cause, such as bereavement; but on other occasions, the insomnia might be the first thing the patient notices. Stress and depressive illness often go hand in hand. Depression hits many people from all walks of life at some point in their lives – and the oddest thing about it is that the condition isn't always obvious to the sufferer, and doesn't always make him or her feel unhappy. Apart from insomnia, the symptoms can be very varied, and include loss of energy, and lack of interest, negative thinking, social withdrawal, irritability, guilt, eating too much or too little, etc. Telling a depressive to snap out of it doesn't help at all. Most people who suffer from depression would dearly love to snap out of it and re-enter the world, but find it incredibly difficult. They feel a pain and a burden to their nearest and dearest – hence the feelings of guilt which only exacerbate the depression.

Many cases of anxiety and depression can be effectively treated with various forms of therapy including drugs, counselling, and support groups. As the underlying condition responds to treatment, so does the insomnia.

In some cases, although exact numbers are not known, the insomnia is not secondary to any other disorder, but intrinsic. (This is also known as 'primary' insomnia.) This condition has only recently been recognised, and some doctors are beginning to think that primary insomnia may be rather more common than was previously thought. Sometimes these intrinsic sleep disorders show themselves by very irregular breathing patterns, or unusual behaviour such as sleepwalking. Psychiatrists don't, on the whole, know very much about intrinsic sleep disorders, so if they suspect one they will usually refer the patient to yet another specialist, in a sleep laboratory.

When doctors make a diagnosis, they are trained to identify the main symptoms, consider the possible causes, and then go through a process of examination and questioning until the initially long list of possible causes is narrowed down to one or two 'probables'. These form the basis for further investigation and assessment.

This means that the doctor will ask a series of questions, some of which may seem quite irrelevant, but be patient: they are all designed to rule out possible alternative causes, and to home in on an accurate diagnosis. The best thing you can do to help the doctor is to explain the effect the problem is having on your life, how and when it started, and what makes it better or worse.

Don't be surprised if your doctor diagnoses you as suffering from something other than insomnia. Sleep disorders are such a common side-effect of various medical and psychiatric problems, that doctors tend not to think of insomnia as a condition in its own right. Instead, they are predisposed to see it as a symptom of some other, underlying illness, and this will often direct their choice of treatment.

The more help you can give your doctor (preferably a sleep diary along the lines of the one provided in Appendix 1 – or a list of the remedies you have already tried, other symptoms and possible causes apart from your physical health), the better equipped your doctor will be to help you.

Obviously, medical and psychiatric conditions require appropriate treatment. Alternatively, if bereavement, redundancy, divorce or other stressors turn out to be an important cause of the insomnia, counselling may be the answer and this is often the next stage of the insomniac's progress through the medical system.

STEP 2 – COUNSELLING

Many people shy away from the thought of consulting a psychiatrist or counsellor – images of straitjackets and emotions gone haywire still dominate our perception of things to do with the mind – but don't panic! Seeking help for stress – and let's face it, we are all prone to stress, and stress is often the root cause of insomnia – is an entirely normal and sensible course to take. You would probably be surprised how many of your friends have sought help in this way, at some point in their lives. The myth that seeking psychiatric help denotes a weakness of character may be preventing them from talking openly about their experiences.

Juliet's Story
'I went through a terrible time with insomnia, and I knew it was stress-related. My father had died, and my

53

marriage was going through a rocky patch. To make matters worse, my little daughter Kate seemed to act out my anxiety – as if she was picking up on the atmosphere. She too wouldn't sleep at night. She started acting like a baby again even though she was eight, and where she had normally been a placid child, she started getting awful temper tantrums.

My GP suggested I saw a counsellor. I must admit, I found the idea daunting. What if I was going mad? The woman I was referred to was incredibly reassuring. After several weeks of weekly one-hour visits, together we pinpointed the root of my anxiety and sleeplessness. I had had a terrible fallout with my father when I was eighteen, and the fact that I hadn't talked about this with him and made amends before his death was haunting me. I reckon I knew that all along, but belittled its importance. I couldn't talk to my husband about it for fear he would think me silly and immature. He was obviously picking up on my lack of communication – we normally do talk about everything – and was feeling resentful, imagining I was concealing far worse things from him. The counsellor got me to write to my father, even though he was dead. In the letter I expressed my regret over our blow-up all those years back, and I told him I loved him. It felt very strange writing it, but also very therapeutic. I also started to talk to my husband again, and he seemed to blossom under the attention! I told a friend all about this, and she said, "Oh goodness, I've been in counselling for months – isn't it brilliant!" Another friend of ours is seeing someone as well – so obviously it's nothing to be ashamed of. Oh yes! And I'm sleeping better too. I've been taught how to manage my stress levels, through exercise, writing, if I feel angry; to face up to my feelings rather than bottling them up – loads of practical suggestions. I wish I had done it earlier.'

So take courage from Juliet's story. If you think stress or depression is affecting your sleeping, talking to someone sympathetic like a counsellor could well be of help. Certainly it is a better course to take than resorting to hypnotics or sleeping pills. Most counsellors see patients for an hour at a time, perhaps once a week. The two of you decide how long these consultations will go on for, but try to stay with it for at least three months. Remember, you are building up a relationship of trust with an independent, professional person – and any relationship takes time to get established. He or she will probably want you to look into your childhood (remember how Sarah's childhood experiences of fearing going to bed affected her adult behaviour?) as well as looking at your present lifestyle and any worries you might have. Fees vary from region to region, and if you are on a low income, you can sometimes negotiate reduced fees. Some organisations suggest that clients make a donation of their choosing after a consultation. Contact the British Association for Counselling for details of counselling organisations in your area. Booklets detailing the organisations can be obtained free from the association, or from your local library. Alternatively, ask your GP for a recommendation.

STEP 3 – THE SLEEP LAB

If you get this far into the system, you'll find that most sleep labs are based in hospitals. In my experience they tend to be staffed by the more eccentric type of clinician, but that is one of the joys of this rather esoteric night out. As the name implies, the purpose of sleep labs is to study you while you sleep – if, that is, you find that the unfamiliar surroundings don't keep you awake all night!

Should you receive an invitation to stay the night, you'll be asked to turn up at the lab in the evening, after most academics and clinicians have gone home. After changing into nightwear, you'll be connected to a number of recording devices; wires will be attached (painlessly) to your head, so that the brain waves can be measured, and other sensors will be attached to other parts of the body. It might sound a bit like an old 'B' horror movie featuring Boris Karloff, but rest assured – this is a bona fide medical procedure. It is a lengthy process, and can take up to an hour, so bring a book. When the wiring has been completed, the monitors will be checked to ensure each separate wire is making a good contact. Then the lights will be dimmed, and you're left alone to sleep.

You won't be entirely alone, however, because the nurse or sleep scientist attached to the unit will be watching you, through an observation window or on closed circuit TV. If you wake in the night, you can get up and walk around – the monitors are portable – and ring for the nurse if necessary.

The number of nights spent in the sleep lab may vary, depending on the nature of the sleep problem, and after this, all the information will be assessed by the sleep scientist and relayed to your GP, who will discuss it with you.

The procedure is expensive, and not everybody is going to be sent for such an intensive assessment – and even for those who are, it's no magic cure. However, some insomniacs have been helped merely by finding that the tests showed that they slept far longer than they thought they had. This was in itself very reassuring, and enabled them to stop worrying so much about not being able to sleep – which improved their sleeping performance!

If a breathing problem is diagnosed in the sleep lab, the patient will then be referred to a department of respiratory medicine for further tests and treatment.

Now that we've followed the insomniac's progress from GP through counselling and into the sleep lab, which is really the last resort, let's go back to the doctor's surgery and take a look at a cure which should not be ruled out in the short term: hypnotics, or sleeping pills.

Reference

British Association for Counselling
    37a Sheep Street
    Rugby
    EV21 3BX
    tel: 0788-578328

CHAPTER 12

Sleeping pills

In the short term, a mild sleeping pill or sedative can help to re-establish good sleeping patterns, though many prefer some of the 'alternative' approaches which I suggest further in the book. Certainly sleeping pills have always been popular. In the old days they used opium, alcohol or the renowned Mickey Finn – a potent (and dangerous) mixture of chloral hydrate and alcohol. None of these was perfect. Opium is addictive, and as if that wasn't bad enough, it causes severe constipation. Alcohol is a central nervous system depressant, and while it does depress the brain sufficiently to help induce sleep, it also causes early morning waking with a sort of rebound anxiety, almost like a spring that has been compressed being allowed to expand too fast. And chloral hydrate is too toxic to be widely used.

Then came those sixties' stand-bys, the barbiturates; but rather like the first lot, these act by depressing the brain rather than promoting true sleep. They too are addictive, and cause tolerance – that is, ever larger doses have to be used to get the same sedative effect. They're dangerous too, and have since been withdrawn from the hypnotic market altogether.

BENZODIAZEPINES

The next generation of sleeping pill or hypnotic, and the one that is still most widely used today, was the benzodiazepine group. The first benzodiazepine was actually

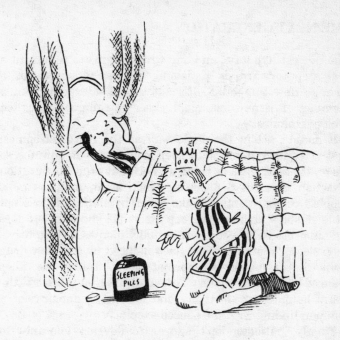

COMING OFF SLEEPING PILLS

synthesised back in the 1930s, but the drugs weren't used in clinical practice until the sixties. It would be fair to say that they revolutionised hypnotic therapy; they had fewer side-effects than the earlier drugs, were less toxic in overdose, and they are reasonably effective. Depending on their speed of action, they are either used as anxiolytics (chlordiazepoxide, diazepam, lorazepam) or for sleep induction (nitrazepam, lormetazepam, temazepam, triazolam). But they still have problems, and fall short of the ideal.

They can cause memory impairment, and in some cases, result in the sudden and unexpected release of aggression.

There is always the danger of dependency. (See address for CITA on p144.)

THE NEXT GENERATION

The newest hypnotic, and one which seems to represent a real step forward, is zopiclone; a strange name, for a strange new compound. It's not a benzodiazepine, but a member of a new chemical class of compounds called cyclopyrrolones.

It doesn't act in the same way as the benzodiazepines; firstly, it gets patients off to sleep in about 20–30 minutes, so it's pretty fast, without being a knock-out drop. Its duration of action is about 6–8 hours, which again matches most people's requirements. Unlike other hypnotics, it does not damage sleep architecture; reports so far show that it does not suppress REM sleep, and actually increases restorative, deep sleep. In other words, sleep induced by this new drug looks pretty much like normal sleep, unlike the sleep induced by other hypnotics. Tests indicate that there is little, if any, hangover the next day, and no memory impairment, a common finding with the benzodiazepines.

Finally, patients don't appear to develop tolerance to zopiclone; there don't appear to be any withdrawal effects, and no reports of dependence or ensuing anxiety.

In short, the early data suggest that this might be rather close to the ideal sleeping pill. The clinical trials with zopiclone, which have involved over 30,000 patients so far, augur well.

However, there have been one or two reports of people on zopiclone who developed symptoms which might suggest a dependence problem; although, to be absolutely fair, these mostly occurred in people who already had a history of benzodiazepine and other drug abuse.

COMING OFF THE PILLS

Sleeping pill dependence is an insidious problem, because it's not obvious. The first signs of drug dependence are usually only noticed during withdrawal. If you have been relying on sleeping pills for a number of years, and the thought of doing without them altogether seems pretty daunting, it may be that you have developed a dependency on them. Firstly, let me emphasise that this is nothing to be ashamed of. People get dependent on coffee, cigarettes – and even, in some cases, carrots(!) – so it is quite understandable that your body should have got used to relying on sleeping pills if it has been fed a diet of them for several years.

Coming off sleeping pills is not necessarily as difficult as you might think. The first thing to do is to enlist the support of your family and your GP. Doctors will readily prescribe a smaller quantity of pills, and you can cut down your intake gradually over a period of 3 or even 4 months. During this period, you should cut down on caffeine and late-night meals, and try to take more exercise and do comforting, positive things for yourself, like taking a hot bath, a weekly massage, or a course of relaxation exercises. On those days when you feel particularly relaxed, try not to take a pill and if you don't sleep, remember that your body is at least rested, relaxed and warm. Self-help organisations like Narcotics Anonymous recommend adopting a 'day at a time' attitude, which makes perfect sense. Rather than think to yourself, 'I'm never ever going to be able to take another sleeping pill,' you tell yourself, 'Just for today, I will choose not to take a sleeping pill.' A day is a manageable concept – if you fail tomorrow, you have at least succeeded today, and you can try again the following day. Once you have had one successful night's sleep without taking a pill, you will feel immensely encouraged to continue. If you don't sleep on another night, try to examine what caused that sleeplessness. Were you hyped up, or worried about anything? Had you drunk too much coffee? Or gone to bed on a full stomach? What made you succeed that other night? Keep a check-list of successes and failures, and that way you can pinpoint what helps you to sleep and what stops you sleeping.

Reference

Narcotics Anonymous
  tel: 071-498 9005
  Service Office (Literature Sales)
  PO Box 1980
  London N19 3LS
  tel: 071-272 9040

CHAPTER 13

The better sleep programme

Well begun is half the battle, or something like that, and if you're determined to win the sleep war, it's essential to start by establishing an optimal sleep pattern. (Optimal, in scientific sleep circles, means falling asleep soon after retiring, and regularly.) The following programme can help considerably, increasing your confidence about getting to sleep, and making bedtime a less anxiety-producing situation.

So, onwards and up the wooden stairs to Bedfordshire, as Mum used to say in the days when Bedfordshire still existed.

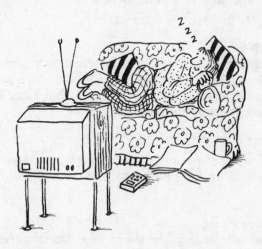

THE BETTER SLEEP PROGRAMME

TWELVE STEPS TO A BETTER SLEEP

Step 1. Exercise
Take more exercise during the day. It really does help you sleep – and sleep better too, as there is good evidence that physical activity causes an increase in deep Stage 3 and 4 sleep. If your routine means that you can't take any exercise until late in the evening, keep it gentle. Nothing too exhilarating, which would have exactly the opposite effect. But remember it's well known that fit people sleep better.

Step 2. Daylight
If possible, try and arrange some exposure to daylight at least once a day. For some insomniacs, this can help to reinforce the natural circadian sleep/wake cycles, and bring them back in line with the day/night cycle. For many of us who work in office blocks or basements where the sun never shines, going walkabout during the lunch hour can help to improve the odds of a good night's sleep. (See also Bright Lights, below.)

Step 3. Naps
No naps during the day at all, however dozy you might feel. A splash of cold water on the face, a brisk walk, a good radio play or a conversation; whatever it takes, but no coffee or tea later than the mid-afternoon.

Step 4. Unwind
Wind down to bedtime. Stop all work and stressful activities about an hour and a half before you plan to go to bed.

Step 5. Bedtime
Go to bed only when you're sleepy tired. Do not go because of habit, and certainly not just because it's the conventional time to retire.

Step 6. Lights Out
As soon as you slip between the sheets, put the light out.

Step 7. TV
Don't read or watch TV in bed – these are waking activities –
even a mind-numbing Open University programme on some
esoteric subject can jog you into wakefulness.

Step 8. Physical Relaxation
Do your relaxing exercises for the first 10–12 minutes after
retiring. If you're practising Progressive Relaxation (see
page 99), take it slowly; don't overtense the muscles, as
relaxation is all about 'letting go'. PR isn't the easiest skill to
acquire, so it's well worth practising the routine at other
times during the day until you've got it right. Alternatively,
you could try completing the exercises last thing before you
go to bed.

Step 9. Mental Relaxation
You've achieved physical relaxation, but if thoughts are still
racing through your mind, don't try too hard to fall asleep.
You can't force it, and straining for sleep is highly counter-
productive, generating nothing more than frustration and a
sense of failure. Remind yourself that sleep will come when
it's ready, and in the meantime relaxing in bed is a pretty
good thing to be doing anyway. Reflect on what sort of day
it's been; and in the words of the song, 'accentuate the
positive, eliminate the negative'. Consider any problems that
have cropped up, and make a note to yourself to do something about them tomorrow. Then remember the good things
that happened, however small. And if new thoughts intrude,
say to yourself, 'I'll deal with that tomorrow.' In other words
– clear the decks for a good night's escapism.

Step 10. Get Up!
If you're still not asleep within twenty minutes, get up. In
fact, you could even get dressed, and get involved in some

sort of activity (but outside the bedroom), until you do feel sleepy. Then it's back to bed, and put that light out!

Step 11. Repeat Step 10
Do this as many times as necessary.

Step 12. Wake Up!
Set the alarm to wake you at the same time every morning. Don't deviate – don't sleep in just because it's the weekend, because then it'll be harder to get to sleep the next night, as your body rhythms begin to drift away from the day/night cycle. If waking up is the problem, get a really loud and offensive alarm clock, and put it just out of arm's reach from the bed. If light or noise is causing early waking, try eyepatches or earplugs respectively.

If you follow the above routine rigidly for several weeks, giving it enough time to 'set', you should find that your sleeping problems are very much less severe, and may have disappeared altogether. This is all about forming good habits, and after you've got the right habits, the occasional deviation won't cause too much trouble, but don't let it become a (bad) habit!

Regularity itself is just as important as the details in the programme, so if you find that there is one particular item in the routine that doesn't work for you, don't despair. Remember it takes all sorts . . . For example, some can only sleep if there is absolute quiet, while others, unbelievable as it may seem, need noise, and can only get off to sleep if the radio is on, or while wearing Walkman headphones. The noisy sleepers are an odd group; they are not affected by late-night coffee drinking, and in fact they find coffee actually helps them to get to sleep! More surprisingly, the same people often say that while at university or college, they were the only ones who fell asleep while taking amphetamines for examinations. Those who require silence are the opposite – late-night coffee disrupts their sleep.

So if you're the type who really needs a little background noise, make that a part of your routine. But if what you want is sensory isolation, then earplugs and eyeshades can make a big difference.

Before I close this chapter, here is one more remedy which has helped many insomniacs. If the sleep programme seems too complicated (it isn't really), or if you prefer a techno-fix, then I heartily recommend . . .

BRIGHT LIGHTS

Light (daylight or artificial) has a profound effect on the sleep/wake cycle (see Chapter 14). For example, if your problem is early waking, try exposure to bright light in the evening. This will increase your alertness, so that you won't feel like going to bed until later than usual. This should ensure that you wake later, at a more convenient time.

A more common problem is that of the night owl, who can't get to sleep at night, and has real problems getting up in the morning. This sleep disorder is caused by an abnormally long circadian rhythm – the bedside clock says it's time to sleep, but your body clock is running late, and insists that you're wide awake, and it's too early for bed. For night owls, the lighting remedy is used in exactly the opposite way than for the early waker. Reset your body clock every morning with a dose of strong white light. This will kickstart the day, and by starting your circadian clock earlier than usual, it will help to ensure that by the end of the day, your body clock will be in agreement with the bedside clock, readying you for sleep.

If your bedroom faces east, and it's a sunny morning, simply throwing the curtains wide may do the trick. But if the sky is overcast, if your bedroom faces the wrong way, and particularly if you suffer from Seasonal Affective Disorder (SAD), then phototherapy, to give it its proper name, is well worth trying. Sufferers of Seasonal Affective Disorder often feel like night owls gone haywire. You have probably read magazine and newspaper articles highlighting the problems of the SAD syndrome – but what exactly makes some of us SAD sufferers? And how can the ensuing insomnia be cured?

SAD sufferers are usually sensitive to reduced sunlight. When light enters the eye, it is transmitted to the pineal gland located at the base of the brain, which secretes melatonin – a powerful hormone which affects sleeping, moods, and seasonal reproductive cycles. If you are a SAD sufferer, melatonin production is happening later at night than usual, resulting in a 'sleep hangover' – and those all-day blues. While most people's body clock mechanism tells them when to sleep and when to wake up, that of the SAD sufferer is somehow short-circuited.

The best cure isn't drugs or even psychotherapy, but good old daylight – the precise commodity which is in short supply during winter months! Phototherapy or light therapy – daily exposure to bright lights – is now used with an 85 per cent success rate to treat the winter blues. You bask in front of a special full spectrum light unit or box first thing in the morning, to kickstart the system, and kid your body that you're lying on a beach in the West Indies. One to four hours' worth of basking is required daily, and don't expect overnight miracles. It does take a while to work its magic. You can use it any time during the day, but avoid last thing at night – unless of course you're planning to boogie till dawn.

Light boxes now start at under £100 and fit neatly under a table or desk. Some are even portable, like the 'Karri-Lite' sold by Full Spectrum Lighting Ltd. Outside In also sell light boxes, which can be placed beside the bed for maximum impact. Unfortunately you have to sit (or lie) about 20 inches from the box for half an hour or so for the phototherapy to work, so you might find the light visor more convenient. This Buck Rogers device consists of a cap with an illuminated visor, powered by batteries. You can potter about the kitchen, getting the breakfast ready or the kids off to school, while getting your dose of light. You might look like an extra from an early sixties science fiction film, but it actually does work. And there's more to it than that, because not only does it cure SAD and the 'night owl' syndrome, there is also increasing evidence that this simple little gadget may be just as effective at treating ordinary depression as well. It might just spell an end to the blues.

References

Full Spectrum Lighting Ltd
  Unit 1
  Riverside Business Centre
  Victoria Street
  High Wycombe
  Bucks
  HP11 2LT
  tel: 0494-448727

Outside In
  Unit 21
  Scotland Road Estate
  Dry Drayton
  Cambridge
  CB3 8AT
  tel: 0954-21195

MIND
  tel: 071-637 0741

SAD: Winter Blues by Dr Norman Rosenthal (Fontana, £3.99)
SAD – Winter Depression and How to Cure It by Angela Smyth (Thorsons, £5.99)

CHAPTER 14

Melatonin

The brain produces, and is influenced by, many different hormones. Melatonin is one of these, which is produced by the pituitary gland at the base of the brain, and is closely linked to sleep patterns. Production of the hormone is suppressed by light, so levels of melatonin in the body are negligible during the day, but after dark, melatonin synthesis goes into overdrive. It's not absolutely clear what melatonin does in humans, but in animals which hibernate it is instrumental in setting the body clock. As the night draws in, and the days get shorter, the amount of melatonin produced by these animals increases. Their metabolic rate begins to slow down; they accumulate body fat, and finally settle down to sleep through the long winter months until spring, with increasing daylight, switches off their melatonin and brings them back to life again.

In human volunteers melatonin has been found to shorten the sleep latency time – that is, the time between going to bed and falling asleep – and so it may find a use as a hypnotic. In the meantime, however, the 'dark hormone' is being used rather more specifically. Jet lag, for example, which disturbs the normal circadian sleep/wake rhythm, can be helped if the jet-lagged subject's clock can be reset; either with bright light at the new waking up time, or by giving melatonin at the new time for going to bed, or both.

As we have seen in Chapter 11, there is a link between sleep and depression too. Depression typically causes early-morning wakening; and prolonged sleeplessness can often trigger depression in someone who is prone to it. Bright light can be used very effectively to treat Seasonal Affective

Disorder, or SAD; and now there is evidence that bright light may be as effective as anti-depressants in treating the common variety, non-seasonal depression as well.

It's almost certainly no coincidence that the incidence of insomnia gets worse as you go north. It's thought that this is linked to the changing length of days and nights: our sleep/wake cycle is tied to the rhythm of day following night, as well as social cues; but when in the summer the daylight lasts for up to twenty hours or more, and in winter it's more or less constantly dark, this can trigger sleep disturbances in vulnerable people.

In some northerly communities the incidence of sleep disturbance is reported to be as high as 40 per cent. There are even reports of mental disturbance linked to abnormally skewed day/night cycles: it is said that in Alaska, the Inuit Eskimos develop a mid-winter syndrome of depression and changes in sleep patterns, which sounds rather like Seasonal Affective Disorder. It is reported to be triggered by lack of light, and cured by flying south or, more conveniently, exposure to intense light.

There have been recent attempts to construct a Grand Unifying Theory of mood, sleep, light and dark, and everything. There is some evidence that the chemistry of melatonin and serotonin, the neurotransmitter involved in both sleep patterns and mood, may be interlinked. Bright light switches off melatonin; melatonin inhibits serotonin formation; therefore, by using bright light to switch off melatonin, serotonin increases – and so does a feeling of well-being.

CHAPTER 15

Yet more remedies

Rest assured, no one ever died of insomnia *per se*, but it's pretty darned unpleasant and, as your doctor might say, there's a lot of it about. Not surprisingly, there's a plethora of alternative and D-I-Y remedies. Some seem to work, others might not be quite so good – but all of them have helped some of the people, some of the time. So here, for the sleepless and the baggy-eyed, are a dozen more low-tech ways of beating those bedtime blues. One of them may be right for you.

TWELVE DO'S AND DON'TS LAST THING AT NIGHT

1. Cigarettes, Coffee and Chinese Food
Avoid stimulants. These include: nicotine (no late-night cigarettes!) and caffeine. There is caffeine in coffee, tea, cocoa, cola drinks, chocolate and over-the-counter painkillers, so check the ingredients. Other drugs which prevent sleep include beta blockers (for high blood pressure), ephedrine (in some anti-asthma medicines and decongestants), and marijuana.

Nicotine patches as well as cigarettes have been implicated in causing insomnia and nightmares. It's difficult to tell whether it's the patches, or cigarette withdrawal (which also causes insomnia), but it seems entirely likely that a constant trickle of nicotine into the blood (especially from the 24-hour patches, the shorter acting patches may be better in this respect) could cause sleep problems.

Late-night Chinese meals can cause problems, because some people are kept awake by monosodium glutamate. The food dye tartrazine can have a similar effect, so avoid orange squash; and also (if you can) avoid arguments, strenuous exercise and work. The only stimulating and strenuous activity which actually encourages sleep is sex, although for some reason this usually works better for men.

2. Have Some Madeira, M'Dear

A little alcohol can help – many people swear by a tot of whisky – but beware of overdoing it. You may get off to

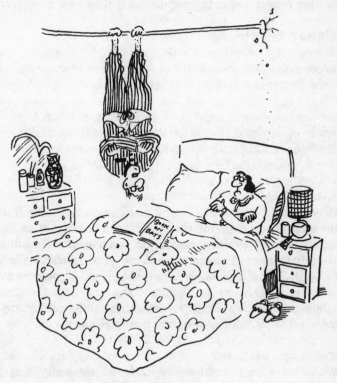

THE CURES

sleep, but the odds are you'll wake in a few hours because the demon drink plays havoc with the sleep rhythms of the brain and besides, who wants to nurse a thumping head in the morning?

3. Milky Drinks

For those who don't approve of alcohol, try a milk and cereal-based drink. Yes, Horlicks or Ovaltine really can help. They contain the amino acid tryptophan, which is converted in the brain to the sleep-inducing chemical serotonin. And if you are worried about gaining weight, look out for the low-fat varieties of milky night-time drinks now available.

4. The Chemistry Set

If you can't stand milky drinks, try the chemical way. Tryptophan (see section 3) can be obtained in capsules, and some find that 1,000 to 1,500mg before bed is very helpful. Others report that inositol (part of vitamin B complex) does the trick, alone or together with 500mg vitamin C and a pinch of vitamin B6. Alternatively, 1,000 to 1,500mg of calcium together with 200–500mg magnesium might help – this is supposed to be good for 'restless legs'.

5. Jus' Juice

Or you could follow the latest American craze. According to the juice gurus, drinking the juice from a mixture of broccoli, tomato, carrot, spinach, asparagus and blackberries will see you off to sleep. Personally, I think putting that little lot through the juice extractor is more likely to keep you awake, and the neighbours as well, but the end result contains vitamin B6, magnesium, calcium and folate, and there is some evidence that these can help induce sleep.

6. Allergic to Sleep?

While we're on the subject of foods, an estimated 1 in 10 people suffer from food intolerance. One of the symptoms is insomnia. If you think you may have a problem try the excellent *Complete Guide to Food Allergy and Intolerance* by Jonathan Brostoff.

7. Sweet Dreams

If you suffer from bedtime hypoglycaemia (symptoms include hyperventilation, a pounding heart and high anxiety), finish the day with a wodge of stodge. A roll would do, or you could eat a bowl of oatmeal, which some herbalists claim has a soothing effect.

8. A Green Sleep, in a Green Shade

Back to traditional remedies. Many books of herbal medicine recommend lettuce and celery as mild tranquillisers, and there are traces of a tranquillising chemical in both of these vegetables. If you like a green salad, this may be for you.

9. Herbs

'I have started sprinkling lavender oil on my pillow at night,' says Paula. 'It is strangely very soothing, and together with herbal teas, and Bach flower preparations, like vervain, has certainly helped me get better sleep in recent months.' Herbalists also recommend lavender and hops (both of which can be taken internally or placed under the pillow), and, in alphabetical order, almonds, aniseed, catmint, camomile, cowslip, fennel, Jamaican dogwood, lime, marjoram, may blossom, melissa, mullein, oats, orange blossom, passion flower, poppy seed, rosemary, willow and valerian – the list goes on and on. Try Quiet Life, Neurelax, Passiflora or Kalms, or browsing through a book of herbal remedies.

Traditional Chinese medicine, incorporating herbs, can also help insomnia. A TCM doctor will try to find out the particular cause. Herbs regularly used are fleece flower stem, poria, and wild jujube seeds. The herbs do not sedate the patient, but appear to have a beneficial effect on the nervous system. Sleeping on a gypsum pillow is a familiar Chinese do-it-yourself remedy, and there is an effective acupressure, massage and exercise routine for insomnia. For further details contact The Register of Traditional Chinese Medicine.

And I must mention Gerard House, who sell a very popular preparation called Valerian Compound Tablets which contain valerian and Jamaican dogwood, together with hops, passion flower and the oxymoronic wild lettuce.

10. Oils

Aromatherapists do it with essential oils including basil, bergamot, camphor, camomile, cypress, frankincense, geranium, jasmine, juniper, lavender, mandarin, marjoram, melissa, myrrh, myrtle, neroli, orange, peppermint, petitgrain, rose, sandalwood, thyme, vetiver and ylang-ylang. Aromas have different associations for different people, so choose the one you like. One popular sleep-inducing remedy is 5 drops camomile, 3 vetiver and 2 melissa or lime, to be added to the bath.

11. Homeopathic Remedies

Homeopaths believe in at least eight different types of insomnia, and prescribe different remedies for each. One popular treatment is Weleda's Avena sativa comp.

12. Sound and Light

There are audio tapes available of music which gradually gets slower, helping the brain waves settle down for the night. Health food shops often stock these, or alternatively, colour therapists say putting a blue light bulb in the bedside lamp can help.

A Reminder

Insomnia can be caused by medical problems which must be treated before the insomnia can be cured. The menopause can trigger sleeplessness, which is often alleviated by HRT; depression is a common cause, as are cardiac problems, asthma, and intermittent and chronic pain. See your doctor.

Hypnosis
The Institute of Complementary Medicine has a list of recommended practitioners (071-237 5167).

Transcendental Meditation
For information call the TM organisation free on 0800-269303.

References

Sound Asleep audio tape, available on Carma Sounds (CRS Records).

Valerian Compound Tablets
  Gerard House Ltd
  Wickham Road
  Bournemouth
  Dorset

The Register of Traditional Chinese Medicine
  19 Trinity Road
  London
  N2 8JJ
  tel: 081-883 8431

Complete Guide to Food Allergy and Intolerance by Jonathan Brostoff (Bloomsbury Press, £9.99)

CHAPTER 16

Eat to sleep

One of the most natural ways of improving your sleep, and particularly core sleep, is by taking more exercise. But what if you don't feel like it? Are you too tired? Or lacking in energy? If so, then check your diet.

A poor diet will leave you with a distinct lack of get up and go – and even if you think you eat well, the odds are there's room for improvement. In fact, your doctor has probably never seen a completely healthy, optimally nourished person. In a recent study of forty-five British athletes, carried out by the London-based Institute of Optimum Nutrition, not one was free of nutritional deficiency.

Optimum nutrition is known to improve the efficiency of muscle cells, so the Institute tested the effects of dietary supplements on athletic performance. After three months of treatment, the runners dramatically improved their times over a 25-mile course, and the weightlifters increased their maximum lifts by an amazing 50 per cent. All the athletes felt less tired, more energetic, and recovered more quickly after their events.

But optimum nutrition isn't only for athletes. The increased energy that comes along with improved nutrition is just as helpful for hard-pressed commuters, executives, parents, shoppers and socialites.

THE RIGHT STUFF

Optimum nutrition is a combination of eating the right types of food, and adding the right kinds of supplement – and it starts with cutting down on that demon of dieters, sugar. Sugar in sweets, cakes and other sweet foods is rapidly absorbed into the blood, and causes a swift rise in blood sugar. This triggers a surge of insulin, which knocks the sugar levels down and after two or three hours leaves people feeling tired and hungry.

This pattern, known as reactive hypoglycaemia, is a sure recipe for low energy levels. It is made worse by alcohol, excessive tea or coffee drinking, and smoking – so stub out that cigarette and switch, if you can, to herb teas. Eat more complex carbohydrates; potatoes, rice, pasta and muesli at mealtimes, and snack on nuts or seeds instead of chocolate. These foods give a longer, slower rise in blood sugar which will provide you with healthier, longer-lasting energy.

Stress makes reactive hypoglycaemia much worse, and is a common cause of fatigue. City life is particularly stressful – it is said that more than 50 per cent of city-dwellers experience sustained stress once a day or more. If you have stress symptoms (anxiety, poor appetite, sleeping problems), stress-reducing techniques can be very helpful in improving your energy levels. Try yoga, Transcendental Meditation or simple, straightforward walking. A brisk twenty-minute walk after lunch not only reduces stress, and boosts energy levels, it also combats the afternoon energy dip that many people experience after the midday meal. What is more, exercise is one of the few factors that can improve blood sugar control. It increases the sensitivity of the body's response to insulin, leading to smoother control of blood sugar levels.

Finally, try launching your day with an energy-promoting breakfast. For your delectation, may we recommend: live yoghurt mixed with wheatgerm, mashed banana to sweeten, and a garnish of sesame, sunflower or pumpkin seeds. This is not only tasty, but is also an easy to digest, balanced meal with the right sorts of unsaturated fatty acids.

NUTRITIONAL DEFICIENCIES – AND WHAT TO DO ABOUT THEM

No fewer than thirteen vitamins and minerals are needed to turn glucose (the cell's fuel source) into energy. Even a well-balanced full-calorie diet is unlikely to provide optimal amounts of all of them and to make matters worse, at any one time about one in five people are on a diet. Dieting is an all-too-common cause of low energy, not only because calorie restriction results in a general slowing down of the metabolism, but also because many diets lead to nutritional deficiencies.

So you might like to consider supplementing your daily food intake. In the green corner, there's juicing (drinking mixed vegetable and fruit juices designed to contain the correct combinations of nutrients); and in the scientific corner, there are nutritional supplements in pill form.

The seven most critical nutrients in the energy cycle are vitamins B3, B6 and C; and the minerals chromium, zinc, magnesium and manganese. For pill-poppers, the recommended daily doses are: B3 100mg, B6 100mg, C 1g, chromium 100mcg, zinc 15mg, magnesium 50mg and manganese 3-5mg. This seems like an awful lot of pills to swallow, but you can reduce them to four; two Bio-Antioxidants, one Bio-C and one Bio-Chromium, all from Pharma Nord UK.

If you prefer supplementing your diet the natural way, consider the humble vegetable. Broccoli contains vitamin C, as well as pantothenic acid, iron and folic acid. Carrots are a good source of zinc and manganese, as well as copper and pro-vitamin A. Add apple for chromium, sweet pepper for B6 and a parsley garnish for magnesium, and you have a high-energy natural juice with a refreshingly different taste.

For a daily dose of Green Energy, take 8oz broccoli; 8oz carrots; 12oz apples; 6oz sweet peppers and a 2oz bunch of parsley. Wash all ingredients thoroughly, combine, juice and serve in a tall glass with ice. If you wish, you can add a liberal sprinkle of turmeric, cinnamon or clove, which contain Insulin Promoting Factor. Drink half the juice only for the first week, then increase the dose gradually through the second week. (Always buy fresh, deeply coloured produce. Use organic fruits and vegetables wherever possible, to minimise exposure to pesticides.)

If the above recipe helps, but you'd like to try something a bit stronger, then maybe it's time to move on to some of the more serious stuff. Advanced juicers sing the praises of two plants above all others, namely alfalfa and wheatgrass. Alfalfa is an extraordinary vegetable, with roots that reach down thirty feet or more into the soil, drawing up minerals unavailable to other, shallower-rooted species. Alfalfa juice contains calcium, magnesium, phosphorus, potassium, zinc, iron and silica, and a full range of vitamins including vitamin A, the B group, C, E and even vitamin K analogues. As if that weren't enough, it's also a good source of amino acids. Alfalfa juice mixes well with other juices, so you could simply add 6oz alfalfa sprouts to Green Energy Mark 1 to produced a souped up Mark 2 version. Choose fresh alfalfa sprouts with small green leaves, and use at once or keep in the fridge.

If alfalfa is the queen of juices, wheatgrass is the king. Wheatgrass juice is used not only to boost energy levels, but in the USA it is also widely used as an anti-ageing and anti-cancer treatment. It contains not only a full spectrum of minerals and trace elements, but also a complete range of the anti-oxidant vitamins A, C, B6 and E, together with the free-radical scavenging enzyme Super Oxide Dismutase, and a whole range of other goodies. In fact, wheatgrass is so nutritious that it is the only plant that will keep mice, guinea pigs, cows or sheep alive and well through generations – no other single plant can do this.

However, even the keenest juicer would have to admit that wheatgrass juice doesn't taste too good. It is best mixed with other juices, so to make Green Energy Mark 3, the most potent brew of all, add the juice from 8oz wheatgrass to the mix. Choose fresh, deep green coloured wheatgrass. (The snag is that to produce wheatgrass juice, you need a slow-turning wheatgrass juicer, available from some health food shops and mail order companies.)

A simpler alternative is a new liquid breakfast designed by the Institute of Optimum Nutrition. Called Get Up & Go, it contains 100 per cent of the daily requirements of all known micro-nutrients, fibre and essential fatty acids, and is probably the most complete nutritional supplement available. In fact, just about the only nutrient it doesn't contain is Co-enzyme Q. This is available from health food shops.

Co-enzyme Q (otherwise known as vitamin Q), is the latest pick-me-up to hit the high-tech end of the health food market. This compound, which gained UK Professor Peter Mitchel the 1978 Nobel Prize for biochemistry, is gaining a fascinating reputation. It seems to be especially effective in treating heart failure, but it has also been shown to markedly improve energy levels, and, as a potent anti-oxidant, to slow the ageing process in animal studies. An increasing number of athletes are adding Co-enzyme Q to their daily regimen, and, if you're interested, a three-month trial with this supplement is definitely worth trying. The best formulation, Bio-Quinone Q10, is available from Pharma Nord.

HERBS AND ADAPTOGENS

Although the concept of adaptogens is relatively new in the West, in the Far East they have formed the basis of preventative health care for thousands of years. Adaptogens appear to be able to help the body to deal with stress, and although some of the more extreme claims for adaptogens can be discounted, it is clear that they can help to increase well-being and energy levels.

Two of the best-known adaptogens are ginseng and, confusingly, Siberian ginseng. Despite the similar names, the two plants are completely different species, and contain different active ingredients. Ginseng is reputed to improve mental and physical performance, to gradually move a person to his or her physical peak, and generally to increase vitality. Siberian ginseng increases stamina and energy levels depressed by undue demands and stress, and has a growing reputation for increasing resistance to illness.

To these two staples it's worth adding guarana, revered for centuries as the sacred food of the Amazon Indians. Guarana has an undoubted energy-boosting effect. It works a little like caffeine but the effects are much gentler and more sustained, so it should not be taken after midday. It has very little effect on blood sugar levels, and is quite a useful tonic. More traditional herbalists use teas or tinctures of wild oats, vervain, liquorice and skullcap. These are particularly recommended for the treatment of stress-induced fatigue, as they are reputed to have a calming as well as an invigorating effect.

But even this isn't the whole story . . .

FOOD INTOLERANCE

Fatigue and low energy are often reported as an early symptom of developing food intolerance. Symptoms of early-morning tiredness, difficulty in waking up, and feeling lethargic until after noon, should make you suspicious that something in your diet may be wrong for you.

World-renowned expert Dr Jonathan Brostoff, at the Middlesex Hospital in London, believes that exorphins may be involved. These compounds are produced when certain foods are digested, including milk, wheat, maize and barley. But how do you know which food is causing the problem? At least half of all patients with food intolerance experience cravings for the food which makes them unwell, and eat it to excess, because exorphins, which mimic the opiates, have an addictive potential. So, go cold turkey. Stop eating the foods you have a craving for.

If this doesn't work, try a modified exclusion diet. Dr Brostoff finds that some of his patients who complain of excessively low energy respond very well to a no-sugar, no-yeast diet. Try stopping sugar and sugar-containing foods first; and then, if there is no improvement, cut out yeast-based products, fruit, and any foods containing white flour. If even this doesn't work, it may be time to try a full-blown exclusion diet – but this should really be done in association with an experienced allergist, and with the knowledge of your doctor.

There is another form of treatment, but as it's more of a kill-or-cure, it won't appeal to everybody. But it does work . . . it consists of strenuous exercise before breakfast, such as running up and down the stairs or round the block two or three times. The first time will be awful – but rest a few minutes, try again and you'll be amazed how much better you do, and feel. Good luck – and may the force be with you!

References

Institute of Optimum Nutrition
    5 Jerdan Place
    London
    SW6 1BE
    tel: 071-385 7984

Pharma Nord UK Ltd
    Spital Hall
    Mitford
    Morpeth
    NE61 3PN
    tel: Freephone 0800-591756

CHAPTER 17

Meal timing

Breakfast like a king, lunch like a lord and dine like a pauper. There's a good reason for this old adage: regulating your food intake in this way will help to train the body into a better sleep/wake cycle, because food boosts the metabolism, and generally promotes wakefulness. During sleep, metabolism falls by up to a third or even more. (It's circadian rhythms not food that causes the afternoon dip in energy.)

So a hearty breakfast boosts the metabolism, and gets you ready for the rigours of the day ahead. Also, there is evidence that the digestive system is working at its best around this time.

Later in the day, and especially in the evening, the digestive tract begins to slow down. A late dinner may not stop you from falling asleep, but it is more likely to lead to heartburn, indigestion and disturbed sleep. Think how you feel after that late-night curry – not only a full stomach but indigestion too will will keep you tossing and turning and regretting that biryani. An occasional late-night dinner isn't going to do any harm, but if you get into the habit of eating very late, this will certainly increase your odds of becoming a chronically poor sleeper. There is a remedy. In countries where the last meal of the day is usually eaten late, there is the tradition of the promenade, a relaxing evening stroll which helps to settle the system and is part of the winding down process. A slow walk back from the restaurant, if you ate out, or just round the block, if you ate at home, is a good idea.

On the other hand, don't go to bed hungry either, as this makes it more likely that you'll wake with a rumbling stomach, and get into the habit of making early-morning raids on the fridge. And this in turn will tend to make it more difficult to get back to sleep.

Hiatus hernia is a special case. In this condition, the muscle that closes off the bottom of the oesophagus, just where it joins the stomach, is unable to make a tight seal. As a result, food and gastric juices can push up (or reflux) into the oesophagus, causing heartburn and eventually oesoph-ageal scarring. Because the stomach is not sealed off, if a hiatus hernia victim were to attempt a handstand, his or her most recent meal would literally fall out onto the floor. Lying down is the next worst thing, because gravity is no longer helping to keep the food down; so the next large gastric contraction will tend to cause reflux.

The best way to avoid this painful condition is to raise the head of the bed by between 6 and 10 inches, which will also, for completely different reasons, reduce swelling and puffi-ness of the eyelids. In addition, it would be prudent to take some or all of the following precautions:

1. Avoid large evening meals
2. Don't drink too much during the three hours before going to bed
3. Avoid fried foods, and pickles

Drink is important too, and too much of it will lead to nocturnal trips to the loo; especially if alcohol or coffee are on the menu, as both of these are diuretics, and increase the formation of urine. Combined, as they often are in middle-aged and elderly men, with a prostate problem, they are a recipe for a very broken night. In women, the nearest equivalent problem is cystitis. The chronic irritation and burning, and the desire to urinate, is bad enough during the day, but can be a real problem at night.

Cutting back on fluid intake is not the answer, as it is bad for the general health and, in women in particular, increases the risk of urinary tract infections such as cystitis. As a rule of thumb, anything between a pint and half a pint of fluid before bed is about right. This could be either a milk-based cereal drink such as Horlicks, or if you prefer, a glass or two of a herbal tea such as camomile or lime. Fruit juices are fine for most people, unless you are taking a potassium-sparing anti-hypertensive drug such as spironolactone.

A PROGRAMME FOR INCREASED ENERGY, AND BETTER SLEEP

This regime will not only make you feel better, with significantly increased energy levels and improved sleep patterns – it has also been shown to slow down vital aspects of the ageing process.

1. The Vitality Diet

Avoid sugar, refined carbohydrates including white bread, biscuits, cakes and other refined foods, coffee, tea and tobacco. Limit alcohol. Eat more beans, lentils, nuts and wholegrains, more raw or lightly cooked vegetables, and foods high in Omega 3 fatty acids, including oily fish such as tuna, bluefish, herring or squid. For dessert, eat at least three pieces of fruit a day. Drink plenty of water and fruit juices. Supplement your diet with beta carotene, vitamin C, pantothenic acid, vitamins B3 and B6, chromium, zinc, magnesium, manganese and Co-enzyme Q.

2. A Bit of Aerobics

Exercising as little as twenty minutes three times a week will boost your metabolic rate during and after the period of exercise. Ideally, the exercise should be sufficient to raise your heartbeat to 80 per cent of your maximum heart rate (which is 200 beats per minute minus your age in years) and keep it there for at least 12 minutes. Jogging, swimming, cycling, brisk walking and exercise classes are all excellent in this respect.

It's perfectly possible to maintain your strength and stamina through the decades, if you keep up a programme of moderate exercise. It's not only de-stressing and slimming, but life-extending too – we weren't designed to lead a sedentary lifestyle. Dr Stephen Webster, of the British Geriatric Society, says: 'A 60-year-old who exercises regularly may retain up to 80 per cent of the strength and stamina he or she had at 25.'

3. A De-stressing Technique

Stress is one of the most important causes of over-rapid ageing. 'Worriers age more quickly,' says Dr Webster, 'and someone with worry lines etched in their face almost certainly has prematurely old arteries.' Learn one of the many de-stressing techniques. And while we're on the subject of de-stressing, keep on having (safe) sex: one of the common factors found in slow agers is an active sex life.

CHAPTER 18

Sex and sleep

NICKY'S STORY

'There's no doubt about it – sex can really help me sleep.
The trouble is, men are conditioned into not rolling over
and falling into a snoring heap, but that is what I feel like
doing. If I delay that wonderful sleepy feeling, then the
chances are I will be awake all night. Luckily, Sally, my
wife, is pretty understanding. She doesn't have a choice
really. Either she has me snoring away, or tossing and
turning beside her!'

Sex is one of the best ways to get to sleep. It is (or it should
be) fun, and exhausting. Unfortunately, in our over-
crowded and over-stressed environment, sex is often
shelved. Headaches, feeling too tired, disinterest after
childbirth or after disappointments at work – there are a
hundred reasons why our initial ardour so often cools. So a
perfectly good sleep-inducer goes by the board – and once
things get to this stage, resentment and performance
anxiety can kill off what's left of the libido, and turn the
bed from an erotic zone into a no-go zone.

Sexuality is a complex and sensitive thing, and the lack
of desire can have many different causes. It may simply
reflect the sad fact that the one-time object of desire has
lost his/her charms – perhaps s/he's run to seed, developed
too many bad habits, or overstepped the mark once too
often. If it's not beyond mending, it can help to bring the
bone of contention out into the open – if you haven't
already done so. If the issue is too painful you should

consider a counselling service, as the presence of a non-judgemental third party is often helpful in encouraging open discussion.

PSYCHOSEXUAL

The consensus view among psychosexual counsellors is that most cases of low or reduced libido are due to: *harmful early influences*, such as ideas received from one parent or other that sex is unpleasant; *anxieties*, where one person (often the woman) might be worried about her partner, or frightened of him; or *low stimulation levels*, otherwise known as boredom. Counselling is directed towards uncovering which of these factors is involved. Often the problem is compounded by poor communication, so both partners are encouraged to share their frustrations and fears, desires and goals.

NOT TONIGHT, DARLING

Look in the back of most newspapers and you'll find small ads offering help to men suffering from low sex drive. You won't find offers of similar help to women, which seems unfair, as women can also experience periods of low libido. Society puts much more pressure on the male to be virile, so he's far more likely to think of his symptom as a problem, and run for help, than is his partner. But sometimes she needs help too.

Libido is often lessened when the relationship hits a bad patch, or when one partner or the other (but often the man) is just not being thoughtful enough. Other common causes include gross insensitivity, or anatomical ignorance. Communication, or counselling, is the way forward.

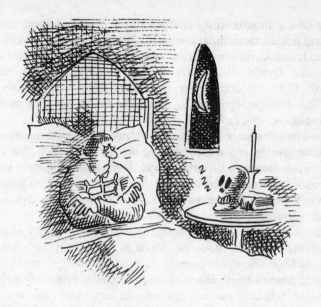

TO SLEEP OR NOT TO SLEEP

MEDICAL

Some cases of decreased sex drive have purely medical causes. Thyroid insufficiency, for example, can squash the libido to almost zero. Treat the underlying medical malfunction, and a whole range of symptoms, including the sexual ones, disappear. Hormonal changes associated with the menopause are a more common cause of low libido, and the most effective way of reversing these is HRT. But it's not just oestrogen; the main libido-determining hormone, in men and in women, is testosterone. In some men, and women, a fall in sex drive is caused by low levels of testosterone – and here, testosterone replacement therapy, available from some private clinics and hospitals, can help.

Although testosterone replacement therapy is extremely effective when used appropriately, it should only be administered by professionally qualified personnel. In one notorious case, a couple turned up at a private clinic with the husband complaining of his wife's lack of interest in sex. She agreed, reluctantly, to be screened; and it turned out that her testosterone levels were indeed on the low side – but not low enough, in the consultant's opinion, to merit replacement therapy. They left empty-handed.

Two months later the husband returned. He had somehow obtained testosterone tablets, illegally, and had been putting very large doses in his wife's food. Her sexual appetite had increased dramatically, to the point where he was finding it difficult keeping up with her. She had begun to grow a moustache, and had become so assertive that he was no longer able to cope. He felt sexually inadequate, guilty about deceiving her, and was convinced she was having affairs with at least two other men.

At this point he decided to confess his sins. Unfortunately, in addition to his poor moral sense, he was a bad tactician. If he had allowed the effects of the tablets to wear off before owning up, the story might have had a less dramatic ending. As it was, his wife was still under the influence of the unofficial testosterone therapy when he broke down and admitted all. In the ensuing argument she beat her husband severely, wrecked much of the family home and trashed the car. No charges were filed.

What he had forgotten, if he ever knew, was that testosterone not only regulates sex drive, but aggression too. High testosterone men in the higher socio-economic groups tend to be high achievers; dynamic, forceful, and often difficult to get on with. High testosterone men who didn't have the benefits of job opportunities or a good education often drift into a life of crime; they have the same drive, but fewer options to use it constructively.

Testosterone has similar effects in women. In one American study, the researchers examined the inmates of a notorious women's prison. They measured their blood testosterone, and then looked to see whether the hormone levels had any relationship to the women's status in the jail and the nature of the crimes they had committed.

The highest testosterone levels were found in the 'top dog'; the next highest in her main supporters, and so on down the pecking order. The lowest were found in the unfortunate women at the bottom of the pile. The researchers then went through the files, checking on the degree of violence associated with sentencing, and found that the 'top dog' inside the jail, with the highest testosterone levels, had also been the most violent criminal. She had returned home one day to find that her husband was asleep, and had not prepared her usual evening meal. She beat him up, destroyed the living room, grabbed a shotgun and went to find her hubbie, who had by now locked himself in the bathroom. She blasted the door down, filled him with lead, and then used the gun as a club to complete the destruction of the bathroom suite. Then she smashed the gun. Then she set fire to the house.

The moral of this story is, caution! Testosterone is marvellous stuff, but don't overdo it.

LIFESTYLE

Hormones are not the end of the story. There are many other factors which can affect desire. Perhaps the best known of these is booze. Alcohol does nothing to increase libido, but can temporarily remove inhibitions, leading to increased sexual activity. (Too much of the stuff makes both partners incompetent, and eventually him impotent.) Lack of exercise lessens desire – but don't start running marathons, as the hormonal changes caused by serious athletic training kill the sexual appetite stone dead.

Again moderate exercise can help, giving quite the opposite effect. Swimming, in particular, has put a sparkle in many a woman's eye. Preposterous? Dr John Moran, a well-known psychosexual consultant based in London's Harley Street, thinks not. 'Swimming twice a week definitely gives the libido a boost. The loss of body heat during swimming triggers a surge of noradrenaline into the bloodstream, which tickles the pleasure centres in the brain and makes you feel sexy.'

This explains the otherwise incomprehensible stories about those dedicated men and women who break the ice on frozen rivers and lakes to go bathing on Christmas Eve! There are others, however, who become almost addicted to the noradrenaline rush. These are the compulsive thrill-seekers, the bungee jumpers, and most intriguingly, the devotees of sado-masochism. 'Mild to moderate pain,' says Dr Moran, 'produces the same surge of noradrenaline as cold does, and this is one of the aspects that gets some people involved in the S and M scene. But it goes farther than that, because any sort of aggression can produce noradrenaline. A row has the same effect, and you know how many rows are followed by sex. Some men and women learn this sub-consciously, and use rows as a kind of foreplay.'

And while we're on the subject, consider the sauna. The combination of heat, cold and birch twigs could not have been better designed to raise noradrenaline levels – and what do we associate with saunas, if not sex?

TIME OF YEAR

Let's go back for a moment to the effects of temperature. If cold was critical you'd expect people to feel sexier in the winter – but it's more complicated than that. For one thing there's central heating; and for another, the dim days and long winter nights bring on melatonin, the 'dark hormone'. Bright light brings melatonin production grinding to a halt, but switch the lights off and levels of the hormone shoot up. Melatonin is a calming hormone, which is one reason we prefer to sleep in the dark – and it could also explain why many couples prefer making love with the lights on.

Melatonin is also involved in Winter Depression, or

Seasonal Affective Disorder (see Chapter 13). SAD sufferers have little interest in sex – all they want to do is binge on carbohydrates and sleep, almost as if they were trying to hibernate. Intense light lifts their depression and boosts their sex drive. (Sparrows are surprisingly similar. City lighting allows metropolitan birds to enjoy sex all year round, to the envy of their rural counterparts, who only do it in the summer months.)

The sexiest weather conditions combine cold to boost noradrenaline, and bright light to reduce melatonin. This is an uncommon combination in many cities, but not in the ski resorts, which could explain both après-ski and the legendary reputation of the ski instructor! (And one more thing . . . cold increases sperm counts, so the ski instructor is probably not only more virile than the average bear, but more potent as well.)

If you're no good on skis, take a spring break in Paris. For centuries the town gallants have been in the habit of walking their fiancées in parks where the horse chestnut trees grow. The animal and plant kingdoms use the same sexual attractant pheromones, and horse chestnut blossom reproduces the steamy atmosphere of a bedroom where tumultuous sex has just taken place. The effects are claimed to be rapid, and sustained. Alternatively collect blossoms when well opened, in mid to late May, and store in the freezer. When required, wrap some in muslin (bouquet garni) and leave in the bath. Bathe, and rise refreshed . . .

A shopping list of unlikely aphrodisiacs
First, make sure the problem isn't with you and your partner. If not, try . . .

1. Swimming twice a week.
2. Something scary after dark, such as a good horror movie.
3. Forget mood lighting – turn up the lights.
4. A skiing holiday.

5. Learn a de-stressing technique. Stress reduces testosterone levels, and relaxing brings them back up again.

6. Take zinc and Vitamin B6. Testosterone synthesis requires both of these, and a deficiency in either reduces libido.

7. Herbal treatments may help. The following recipe will increase your noradrenaline levels: 4g ginseng, 4g kola, 16g saw palmetto and 4g damiana, added to 1 pint boiling water. Leave for thirty minutes, stirring occasionally; strain off liquid, place in fridge. Dose: 25–50 mls, 2–3 times daily.

8. When in Rome . . . the Romans ate lightly cooked animal testicles, made into sausages. Their high testosterone content increased libido in men and women, which made the X-rated bangers very popular. Chronic use was discouraged, as women eventually grew facial hair.

9. If all else fails, try a good bedtime row.

Reference

For marriage guidance advice contact Relate. To find your nearest Relate Centre, look in the telephone directory under 'Relate' or 'Marriage Guidance'. The national office is at:

Herbert Gray College
Little Church Street
Rugby
CV21 3AP
tel: 0788-573241

CHAPTER 19

Pain prevention

Chronic pain is one of the most important causes of sleeping problems. A bad back, a sore throat, a headache or the pain of a more serious medical condition can all keep sleep at bay. There are always painkillers, but quite a few people can't or won't take them. What are the alternatives?

PAIN

Pain can be a blessing in disguise. It is the body's way of telling us something is wrong, a vital message that some-

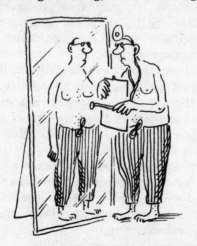

INSOMNIA SELF-CHECK

thing we are doing is injuring us and we had better stop before serious damage is done. Very rarely, children are born with a genetic error that prevents them from feeling pain. They have scarred and burned hands, bruised bodies, broken and twisted limbs – because they never learned not to put their hands in the fire, play with knives or jump from too high walls.

But pain can be malignant and destructive too. Some are plagued with pain with no obvious cause (amputees can suffer from 'phantom limb pain', with pain seeming to originate in a limb they no longer possess), and many more people's lives are made wretched by chronic pain, from arthritis to bad backs to sciatica. So what can we do about pain? How can we reduce its impact on our lives?

What we mostly do, of course, is reach for the medicine cabinet. The Brits take more painkillers than any other nation on earth, not because we suffer more pain but, mostly, it is said, for fear of experiencing pain and losing control. There is a price to be paid for such enthusiastic pill-popping, however, and that is a high rate of gastro-intestinal problems ranging from indigestion to life-threatening ulcers. So, the next time you get a bad back, or a migraine headache, or period pains, don't reach for the pill bottle. Think instead of China.

The Chinese do things rather differently. They pioneered acupuncture as a powerful pain-relieving technique, and still use it very widely. Schoolchildren are taught mental techniques they can use when needed, to enable them to carry on until the pain subsides or until a doctor arrives. Too remote? The SAS use them too. An SAS trainer told me of a young sergeant who broke both ankles while training in the Arctic, but was still somehow able to walk the fifteen miles back to base camp. He used mental pain control techniques to raise his pain threshold, and survive – and so can you.

Try these alternatives to your painkillers.

1. Progressive Relaxation

Next time you get a **tension headache**, or a **sore neck** or **back**, try PR. The more stressed you are, the lower your pain threshold becomes; and clenched muscles, a common response to pain, can make it worse. PR reduces psychological stress, and relaxes the muscles. You'll need a quiet room, so throw out the cat and lock the door. Lie or sit with your eyes closed. Beginning with the toes, tense your muscles for 3 seconds, then relax them for 20 seconds. Repeat: then perform the same routine working up through the major muscle groups, ending with the neck and facial muscles. Try deep breathing; take a slow breath through the nose, counting to 5, then exhale slowly through the mouth while repeating the world 'calm' in your mind.

2. Hypnosis

Hypnosis produces deep mental and physical relaxation, and can suppress the brain's perception of pain. A trained hypnotist talks you into a deeply relaxed state, in which you are more receptive to positive suggestions, such as the hypnotist telling you that the pain is becoming more bearable. This will come in very useful next time you get a **Sunday night toothache!** Also good for **back pain**, and especially **birth pains**. The Institute of Complementary Medicine has a list of recommended practitioners.

3. Massage

Massage relieves the tightening of muscles that can contribute to many forms of pain including **back, neck** and **shoulder pain**. Alternatives to massage include ice packs, heat treatment, stretching routines, exercise, and aromatherapy.

4. Biofeedback

Biofeedback is a higher-tech approach that has only recently become available in a few UK clinics. The Bio bit is to do with training people to control various bodily functions such as heart rate, blood pressure, skin temperature and blood flow through the hands or feet. The feedback element refers to the medical equipment that monitors their progress and tells them how they're doing. Put the two together and you have a powerful technique that has helped many **tension headache** and **migraine** sufferers.

5. Acupuncture

If you're plagued by **arthritis, menstrual cramps** or **facial pain**, acupuncture can help. The original version relies on fine needles placed in the skin at strategic sites. Acupuncturists train for years to learn where these sites are, and what they do.

6. Electro-acupuncture

Electro-acupuncture, a more recent development, has several advantages. Firstly, it does not require needles. Secondly, the better devices locate key sites on the skin themselves. A recent article in the *British Medical Journal* showed this D-I-Y approach to be highly effective in treating **fibrositis**, and there are good reports of electro-acupuncture in treating **dental pain, sprains** and **strains**, **arthritis** and **headache**. There are several home models: *Which Magazine* gave the Acuhealth 900 a very good report. Available from larger branches of Boots, or directly from Acuhealth Ltd.

7. Pain Clinics

Most large hospitals have a pain clinic to help people with chronic or intractable pain. The few cases that do not respond are referred on to one of two centres. Based at St Thomas's Hospital in London, INPUT is a pain management programme which combines medical, behavioural and cognitive methods to treat the untreatable – with very impressive results. The other major centre, at Liverpool's Walton Hospital has recently produced an audio cassette, *Coping with Pain*. The tape is recommended for **arthritis, rheumatism** and **low back pain**; and 75 per cent of people with diseases including **MS, shingles** and **cancer** reported reduced pain, and a more active life or a better night's sleep.

References

The Institute of Complementary Medicine
  tel: 071-237 5167

Acuhealth Ltd
  Freepost (WD 4671)
  London
  W1E 4QZ

Coping with Pain audio tape (£6.25 inc p & p)
  Pain Tape
  PO Box 1
  Wirral
  L47 7DD

CHAPTER 20

Anxiety reduction

If your insomnia is rooted in anxiety, the first step to a
good night's sleep is to learn a good anxiety-reducing
technique; and a good place to begin is where, in all
likelihood, the first overly-anxious men and women began
– with meditation.

MEDITATION

There are many different ways of meditating – for example,
medieval literature refers to fire, water (either running or
boiling) and smoke meditations. In each case the technique
is broadly similar, and involves concentrating on a varied
and randomly changing surface, which is used to take your
conscious mind away from the chatter and worry of daily
existence, and move it onto a transcendental level where
peace and quiet can emerge.

If you prefer to attempt meditation on your own, there
are a number of ways in which you can move towards this
state. You could, for example, if there's no live fire or
running water to hand, concentrate instead on a sound.
Some people do best with sounds which do not obviously
resemble any meaningful word, reducing the risk of free
associating word patterns which could be a distraction.
However, everyone is different, and there are many paths
to enlightenment. Traditionalists might wish to stick with
the sound 'Om'; but many people find they do very well
with words like 'harmony' or 'oriole'.

Whatever the word, and whether it makes sense or not,

the procedure is as follows: find a reasonably quiet room, with a comfortable chair. Sit down, close your eyes, and begin to repeat the word to yourself. In the beginning you'll probably find that you're sub-vocalising, that is making the mouth and throat movements that go with saying the word – but with practice, eventually that fades. You are left with a series of sounds which echo repeatedly through your mind. If you find your thoughts drifting, don't worry, that's entirely natural; but once you become aware of those thoughts, come back as effortlessly as you can to the word. The important thing is not to strain. Take it very easily throughout, don't force things at any stage – let the word carry you. After twenty minutes or so, open your eyes. Wait a minute before getting up to let the body re-enter the world in easy stages.

You'll find that each period of meditation is slightly different. Sometimes you'll find that you're constantly drifting away from the word; other times you'll enter a deep, quiet space like an underground pool, and the twenty minutes will fly past. All the experiences are valid. If you can manage 2 twenty-minute periods each day, once in the morning before breakfast, and once at night before going to bed, you will probably soon notice an improvement in your sleeping quality. You may even find that although the length of sleep doesn't increase, you still feel more awake and more rested during the day – because meditation is capable of giving the body, and the brain, the deep rest that normally only sleep would produce.

Some people worry that if they become too relaxed, they won't be able to work at the fever pitch that their demanding jobs require. This is the wrong way of looking at things, because a stressed mind is inherently less efficient at solving problems than a relaxed one. By learning to relax, either with meditation or any other de-stressing technique, you become better able to cope, and develop better control over your waking behaviour and sleep patterns.

FLORA'S STORY

'I have trained myself to concentrate on a really relaxing image,' says Flora. 'When I'm in bed and can't sleep, I imagine myself in a hammock somewhere beautiful like the tropics. To my left is the sea. As I breathe slowly and regularly, I imagine the rhythms of my breathing to be the rhythms of the sea – it really helps me relax. It's a technique I learned from a yoga class years ago. The instructor "talked" us through this beautiful image, and it was so effective, I fell asleep. Apparently I was snoring gently and the whole class thought this terribly funny!'

If you find it difficult to achieve meditation on your own, Transcendental Meditation is well worth trying. The TM approach is friendly and generally effective, and once past the first session, easy to accept and practise. Their teachers know the ropes, and should be able to guide you onto the meditational path without too much effort.

In some people, however, levels of stress and anxiety are so high as to make meditation impossible; and before a de-stressing programme can be implemented, they have to learn how to deal with one of the extremes of anxiety, the panic attack.

Reference

TM (transcendental meditation)
  FREEPOST
  London
  SW1P 7YY
  tel: 0800-269303

CHAPTER 21

Panic attacks

MARGARET'S STORY

'When I first experienced a panic attack, I had no idea what was going on. It was all very physical. Firstly, my neck felt tight, like someone was throttling me. At the same time, my heart was beating wildly as if it was going to burst, and I had a cold sweat on my face and hands. There was a ringing in my ears and I felt this terrible sense of a loss of self. I didn't dare tell anyone. I thought I was going mad. It seemed to last for ages, but in fact lasted only about twenty minutes. They came quite frequently after that and always unexpectedly. In public was worst. On the underground, when I was walking over a bridge – this terrible feeling of not being normal, of feeling cut off from the world. Coincidentally, I had started counselling, because there was a lot going on in my life. I eventually told the counsellor what was happening and she told me it was a panic attack. I now see that it was like a kettle left to boil too long, and the lid is jumping about, in that I had repressed so many bad feelings and worries that my body was literally telling me to take action. Talking about my worries helped, and also learning to count slowly and breathe gently, rather than gasp for breath as you tend to want to do. It helped me to have someone hold me as well, until the shakes stopped. I used to pray as well, not that I'm very religious, but I do believe in some form of higher spiritual power, and that really helped. I'm now back on an even keel. I had one attack after a year's respite, and I luckily knew how to cope with it.'

When the going gets tough, even the tough get stressed. Oddly, many people suffering from stress are unaware of it, as one of the first things to go is one's better judgement – so how can you tell if you, or your nearest and dearest is suffering?

Early warning signs typically include insomnia, fatigue, irritability, and changes in eating and drinking patterns. Smokers increase their intake, ex-smokers find themselves lighting up. Tact and diplomacy disappear, relationships suffer. And if stress levels increase further, unsociable behaviour can slip into mental illness.

Some personality types develop a form of depression. Insomnia (again), restlessness, and melancholy predominate. Life seems more difficult, less meaningful; the sufferer retreats from the outside world, and some may perform self-destructive acts or even make a suicide bid.

Others develop an anxiety state, which can culminate in the terrifying experience of a panic attack. The victim experiences palpitations, trembling, sweating, nausea and breathlessness. There is often a tingling in the fingers, toes and lips; chest pain; dizziness and the sensation that the legs are about to give way. In a severe attack the victim may feel he or she is going mad, having a heart attack or even dying. And during these attacks we play an even worse trick on ourselves, because our awareness of time alters. Although most attacks last no more than a few minutes, those few minutes can stretch out into a seeming eternity of fear.

In anxiety states the adrenal glands flood the bloodstream with adrenalin. This raises muscle tension, leading to tremor and muscle pain in the neck, back and shoulders. It also increases the blood pressure, speeds up the heartbeat, and increases our anxiety level. The breathing rate shoots up, leading to feelings of light-headedness and tingling in fingers and toes. When the victim feels all these unpleasant symptoms coming on, anxiety multiplies into a panic attack.

ANATOMY OF THE PANIC ATTACK

The first attack usually happens out of a clear sky, but may form from a sort of blueprint for subsequent episodes. For example, if the first attack occurred in a lift, subsequent attacks are quite likely to occur in lifts too. This is because after the first attack, you may well become afraid of the situation that triggered it. The next time you enter a lift, the fear of becoming afraid emerges and can amplify itself in a sort of feedback loop until a full-blown attack develops.

But if you know how the feedback loop operates, you can abort a panic attack. Even better, you can defuse situations which formerly caused attacks, make them safe, and unlearn the fear.

TREATMENT

★ Panic attacks are usually preceded by certain thoughts or emotions. If you become aware of these warning signs, stop.

★ Remind yourself that even if the worst happens, it's only a panic attack. However bad it feels, it'll blow over – and it won't harm you.

★ Don't panic. Slump at the shoulders and neck, let your arms hang. Take a deep breath in, then exhale fully. Now breathe, slowly and gently, through the nose. Feel your stomach moving in and out with every breath. With the first intake of breath think 'twenty'; with the next, 'nineteen', and count on down to zero. Even the first few breaths make a difference, and within a few minutes anxiety is greatly reduced.

★ Some people prefer a re-breathing technique, which corrects the effects of hyperventilation. Place a paper bag over the nose and mouth. Breathe slowly in and out about ten times. Remove the bag for a few minutes, and repeat if necessary.

★ Avoid caffeine. Excessive coffee and tea drinking can

make matters worse by lowering blood sugar, and triggering the release of more adrenalin. Cut down on sugar, which can also stimulate adrenalin release. Studies by the US National Institutes of Mental Health found that 75 per cent of patients suffering from anxiety and panic disorders had a dramatic increase in anxiety after eating sugar. Chocolate is another suspect; there is some evidence that chocolate can trigger panic attacks in those prone to them, so cut back if you can and the panic attacks may become less frequent.

★ Some people find that calcium supplements (1g a day), plus magnesium (up to 500mg a day) reduce the frequency of panic attacks.

CHAPTER 22

Coping with seasonal insomnia

For some, insomnia is seasonal. They're fine during the winter months, but come the spring and the unholy combination of streaming eyes, a blocked nose and cough makes the bed a most uncomfortable place.

HAYFEVER

August may be a wicked month, but for the 6,000,000 hayfever sufferers in Britain, April, June and July are

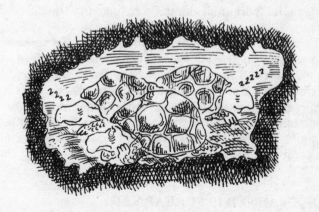

SEASONAL INSOMNIA

far worse. And if it seems that there are more hay-fever sufferers around than ever before, it's absolutely true – the numbers of people with allergic disorders are doubling every ten years, so you, or someone close to you, might well fall victim this summer. All the records were broken in 1992, due to unreasonably high pollen counts. The bad news is that global warming, with the likelihood of longer and warmer summers, will probably make matters even worse.

So what can we do to avoid (or at least minimise) the usual summer problems of streaming eyes, sore throats and running noses? It helps to know which types of pollen are causing your problem, and when they're most likely to be about, so that you can take evasive action. As a rule of thumb, tree pollens are the first to arrive, starting as early as April – so if your symptoms begin around this time, blame the trees. The grass pollens, which are the worst offenders, peak in June and July; while shrub pollens have a longer season. If your symptoms begin in late July or August and continue into autumn, it's more likely to be an allergy to mould spores; while hayfeverish sniffles that carry on all year round (perennial rhinitis) are linked to the house dust mite.

There are exceptions to the above rules. An unexpected encounter with dried flowers, even in mid-winter, can bring on an attack of hayfever; and there are cases of apparent hayfever which are in fact caused by food allergy. This is not common, but can happen when foods cause rhinitis, and the foods concerned just happen to be those eaten most often in summer. (These include strawberries and other summer fruits, orange squash and ice cream.)

FOREWARNED IS FOREARMED

Be prepared. If you know what is causing your problem, you can take evasive action.

1. Start by checking with a pollen calendar, to see when your particular problem pollen is scheduled to arrive.
2. A month or so before P-Day, consult your doctor. Some of the medications prescribed for hayfever take weeks to build up their protective effect, so it's well worth making a pre-emptive strike, rather than waiting until your symptoms begin.
3. As soon as your favourite pollen arrives (and you'll know when it does), call CLARITYLINE on 0800-556610. This 24-hour freephone line will give you the day's pollen count, plus a forecast for the next 3 days.
4. Pollen levels are highest in the morning when pollen is released, and in the evening, when the air cools and the pollen settles again.
5. During the day the pollen count is lowest at ground level – so close upper windows, especially in tall buildings.
6. If you're driving in the country, or through parkland, close the windows and switch off the ventilation system – unless you're lucky enough to be driving a car with pollen filters.
7. Plan your holidays with care! Avoid rural idylls, head for the beach instead as sea air is usually pollen-free.
8. Sunglasses may help to keep some pollen out of the eyes; washing your face and hands after coming in from outdoors may help too.

TREATMENT

If your main problem is sore and streaming eyes, eye drops containing an anti-histamine and decongestant can offer temporary help. Regular Opticrom drops or ointment can be very effective, but should be started a month *before* the hayfever season begins.

If it's the nose that's causing the bother, your doctor is likely to recommend a spray containing either sodium cromoglycate or a corticosteroid. Again, these should be used regularly, and started a month early. (Nasal decongestants can clear a blocked nose, but long-term use can actually make matters worse.)

For widespread symptoms, the solution might be an anti-histamine. These are perfectly good drugs, but do read the instructions in the pack, and tell the GP if you are taking any other medication. Desensitisation is now seldom used. It is not always effective, and is potentially dangerous.

There has recently been a new approach to nasal allergic symptoms, which seems promising. It's a plant-based powder called Nasaleze which you spray into the nose, where it forms a gel-like layer, protecting the nasal tract and sinuses from pollen, house dust and other allergens, without causing sedation. One puff is claimed to provide effective relief for up to 24 hours; so if you suffer from sneezing fits, a blocked nose and all the misery of streaming and itchy eyes, Nasaleze is definitely worth trying.

There are reports that large doses of vitamins C and B6, together with the minerals zinc and calcium, have a protective effect. A similar mix, but with the addition of vitamin B5, is said to reduce symptoms once they've begun. I would be very interested to hear from anyone who has tried this approach.

Finally, it's important to be born at the right time of year, though this is something you obviously have no control over. Exposure to allergens during infancy increases the risk of developing allergies during later life, which is why babies born in the spring, when pollen counts are high, are more likely to develop hayfever or asthma as they grow up. There's not much we can do about this for ourselves, but allergic parents can definitely do something for their babies; namely, arrange it so they are born between September and February! And on a more practical note, protect them as far as possible from cigarette smoke, fur and feathers, house dust, and traffic fumes.

(The first year is critical, as after that babies become less vulnerable.)

References

Nasaleze
  Lark Pharmaceuticals
  36 Haven Green
  London
  W5 2NX

CLARITYLINE (for pollen information)
  tel: 0800-556610

CHAPTER 23

Allergies and asthma

Allergies can contribute to snoring by causing swelling of the mucous membranes of the mouth, throat and airways. They can also cause asthma. If the poor sleeper is known to have allergies, or has asthma, hayfever, conjunctivitis or contact dermatitis, the role of allergens in causing their sleeping problem should always be investigated.

The most common allergens are pollen, animal fur or feathers, and the house dust mite, whose highly allergenic excreta have been implicated in nearly half of all asthmatics. There are many anti-asthma drugs available, but as any good doctor will tell you, an ounce of prevention is worth many pounds' worth of cure. So, to minimise exposure to these allergens, you should ideally aim for a dust-free and mite-free bedroom. This means no deep pile carpets, minimal fabrics, no pets and regular hoovering with a Medivac or Miele vacuum cleaner with special filters. Alternatively, an ioniser next to the bed will knock down much of the dust, and can often be very helpful.

The role of central heating is crucial, as warm bedrooms enable the house dust mite to thrive. A cool or cold bedroom will finish them off, so simply turning down the thermostat can sometimes do the trick – although the beneficial effects will take a few months to work their way through. Unfortunately, cold air can make some asthmatics worse, so be cautious, and for the meantime, keep the anti-asthmatic medications at hand.

The other thing that the mites love is humidity. A good dehumidifier will kill them off, and in the long term can result in significant improvements in asthma, and sleep. In addition to providing a breeding ground for mites, a damp bedroom also provides ideal conditions for certain moulds to grow, moulds which produce clouds of fine, airborne spores which are another common cause of allergies. Here, too, the dehumidifier scores points. However, some asthmatics are intolerant of dry air, so once again, proceed with caution. However, if the mites were the main cause of the problem, their removal will allow the airways to become less inflamed, and the sufferer will in time be better able to withstand cold and dry air.

There are one or two more strategies worth considering. Anti-mite sprays are sometimes used, but the effects are temporary. An alternative is to use micro-permeable bedding, made of Gore-Tex and sold as Intervent by major chemists. This new approach has been shown to be very effective in many cases, but the bedding is expensive; a full set of pillow cases, mattress and duvet covers will cost up to £300 for a single bed.

Finally, food allergies can also play a part in causing sleep problems. For further details, see the excellent *Food Allergy and Intolerance*, by Jonathan Brostoff and Linda Gamlin.

References

Food Allergy and Intolerance by Jonathan Brostoff and Linda Gamlin (Bloomsbury Press)

CHAPTER 24

Cold wars – sleeping through the sneezes

Perhaps you sleep perfectly well through the spring and summer, and only get into trouble when the weather begins to get cold? For you the cause of this seasonal sleeplessness isn't hayfever, but common coughs and colds. It's hard to sleep when you can't breathe, and your throat and head are aching. Do you get colds from December through to April? And would you like to do something about it? Then read on . . .

The average person gets three to four colds every year. The Victorians suspected germs, and tried all sorts of remedies from stuffing the pillow with peeled onions (not recommended unless you want to smell like a greengrocer's) to spraying the bed with carbolic acid, but none of them worked – not even wearing red flannel underwear, widely recommended by health experts at the time.

These days everybody knows that colds are caused by viruses. If there was only one virus, we'd develop immunity after the first cold and then never get another (like measles). Unfortunately, there are hundreds of different strains of virus, and as soon as we develop immunity to one strain another one comes along.

The cold virus usually affects the nose and throat – that nasty blocked state where your head feels like a swollen throbbing football (head cold), but can spread down into the larynx (laryngitis) and lungs (bronchitis). The infection typically lasts between 3 and 6 days, or longer if bacteria

116

invade the infected tissues and set up a secondary infection.

The virus is spread by droplet transmission (coughs and sneezes, as they say, really do spread diseases), and by physical contact. So if you're unfortunate enough to have a cold, there's a lot of sense in putting a hand over your mouth, using a handkerchief, and washing your hands to avoid passing your cold on to others.

If you don't have a cold, avoid the company of those who do. But that's more easily said than done, so what else can you do? I said that colds are caused by viruses – but that's not completely true. What causes a cold is the failure of your immune system to deal with the viruses, and so the first thing to do is to make sure your immune system is working properly.

Fatigue, stress, depression, and not getting enough of certain key nutrients can all affect the immune system – and when the immune system isn't up to par, any viruses around get a clear shot at you. But if you're getting enough rest, feel confident and strong, and eat an adequate diet, you're far more likely to remain cold-free. Also, don't smoke (smokers get more colds, and worse ones), and wash your hands frequently to prevent hand-to-mouth transmission of the virus.

Which brings us to vitamin C. Last year Dr Elliott Dick and his colleagues at the University of Wisconsin took sixteen healthy volunteers and gave eight of them 2g of vitamin C daily, in four doses of 500mg. The other eight received placebo pills. After three weeks of treatment, the volunteers were put in a dormitory full of other people who already had bad colds. Imagine the noise of all that sneezing and wheezing! The vitamin C group caught just as many colds as the placebo group, but their symptoms were much less severe. Coughs fell to a third, sneezes were cut in half, and nose blowing was reduced by a third. Interesting stuff, even if it does sound like something out of Professor Brainstorm!

Dr Richard Passwater, author of *The New Supernutrition*,

believes that colds can be stopped with vitamin C. 'When I feel a cold coming on I stop it in its tracks by taking 2g of vitamin C immediately, then 1g every hour until I go to bed – and that's the end of it.'

Other doctors remain sceptical, but I used to get several colds every winter which would inevitably go down into the chest, leaving me with bronchitis. In 1986 I started taking 1g of vitamin C a day, and since then have had only a few minor head colds, and no bronchitis at all.

But if the worst happens, and you don't believe in vitamin C, what else can you do? The typical cold remedy contains a mild painkiller, which also helps to reduce a temperature, a decongestant, and an anti-histamine, which some people believe can help to reduce allergy-like symptoms such as streaming eyes. Don't take more than one remedy as many contain similar ingredients, and combining them could cause an overdose situation. Drink lots of fluids (non-alcoholic variety).

You might feel like death, but it's generally not necessary to call the doctor unless you develop any of the following symptoms: coughing up green sputum or blood, breathlessness, wheezing, croup, chest pain or blueness around the lips.

REMEDIES

There are over thirty medicines on the market, from Actifed to Vick Vapour Rub. Try until you find something you're happy with. (Antibiotics won't work, because they can't touch viruses, although they can be useful if there is a secondary bacterial infection.)

For the herbally inclined, there are a host of proprietary garlic preparations which many people rely on. And no – you don't smell like a French gourmet chef or look like a potential victim of Count Dracula. Garlic preparations for medicinal purposes are thankfully odourless. For those who believe in homeopathy, there is aconite, gelsemium, Merc. Sol. and Nat. Mur.

Reference

The New Supernutrition by Dr Richard Passwater (Pocket Books)

CHAPTER 25

General health and sleep

We've sorted out hayfever, and coughs and colds. Now let's set about reducing your chances of getting ill. Almost any illness will cause insomnia, because most illnesses tend to disrupt normal sleeping patterns. A healthy body will sleep better than an unhealthy one.

THE IMMUNE SYSTEM

The immune system is a highly complex and many-layered defence mechanism, designed to protect us against the teeming hordes of micro-organisms (bacteria, viruses, parasites) that see us as food and shelter. The system's outer defences consist of millions of free-ranging cells which circulate through the whole body, always on the lookout for invaders. These cells are pumped round the body in the bloodstream, but drain back to the heart via the lymphatics, a system of small vessels rather like veins that drain back through lymph glands in the neck, groin and under the armpits before emptying back into the bloodstream.

If the cells spot an invading bug as they go their rounds, they bring it back to the lymph glands; and there, other immune cells swing into action. They multiply (which is why swollen lymph glands are a sure sign of infection), and release antibodies. These are special molecules that act like guided missiles, looking for the bugs and, once they've found them, sticking to them like glue. This is enough to stop some invaders altogether, but the immune system has another trick up its sleeve; the combination of 'bug plus stuck-on

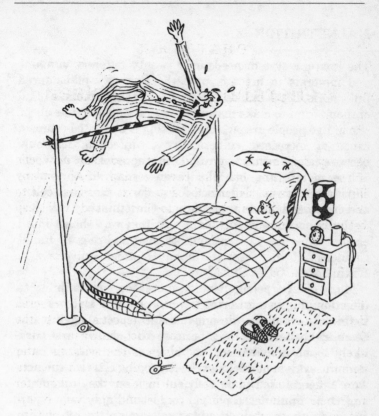

SLEEP AND EXERCISE

antibody' brings the killer cells running. They zoom in on the invading organisms, and gobble them up. End of invasion.

You might think that nothing would get past these defences – and most of the time, very little does. Most of the time, despite living in an environment full of potentially disease-causing organisms, we remain free of infection. There are some bugs, of course, which are so virulent that they seem to be able to break through our defences, or sabotage them – the AIDS virus is a case in point. But there are other areas of potential weakness.

121

MALNUTRITION

The immune system needs over twenty different vitamins and minerals to function properly. Even a well-balanced full-calorie diet is unlikely to provide optimal amounts of all of them – and to make matters worse, at any one time about one in five people are on a diet. Dieting is an all-too-common cause of increased vulnerability to infection, not only because calorie restriction results in a general slowing down of the metabolism, but also because many diets lead to specific nutritional deficiencies – so don't start that celery and crispbread diet in the run-up to Christmas!

The importance of adequate nutrition was shown in an elegant experiment carried out last year by Professor Ranjit Chandra, at the respected John Hopkins University in Baltimore.

Many elderly people have an increased susceptibility to infection, due to a faltering immune system. Doctors used to think that this was an unavoidable aspect of ageing; but Chandra believed it was because the elderly are more likely to be deficient in the minerals and vitamins the immune system needs to work effectively. His test subjects were indeed found to be deficient in many key nutrients, and their immune responses correspondingly below par. He gave them a daily nutritional supplement; within twelve months their immune systems had perked up. Moreover, medical records showed their days off sick had been reduced by an amazing 50 per cent. Professor Chandra predicts that the benefits of supplementation will be just as great in the young, athletes, anyone on a diet, and just about everybody else.

The Chandra supplement has been patented, but isn't yet on the market. In the meantime, visit your health food shop and try Bio-Antioxidant from Pharma Nord UK. These pills, which cost about £8 for a 3-month supply, contain a full range of antioxidant vitamins and minerals vital to the immune system's normal functioning.

SMOKING

Smoking is definitely a problem, as it hits the immune system hard, with potentially devastating results. In the airways, it harms the immune cells which normally protect us against the inhaled micro-organisms that cause coughs, colds, sore throats and bronchitis. This is why smokers are more prone to all these illnesses; but more worryingly, tobacco smoke damages immune cells elsewhere in the body too. This is why smoking is associated with an increased risk of cancer, not just of the lungs, but also the mouth, larynx, oesophagus, bladder, pancreas and cervix.

STRESS

Let's face it, stress is a common cause of most troubles – illness, depression, lethargy – as well as sleeplessness. When insomnia is sporadic rather than continual, stress could well be the problem. Stress in our busy lives is definitely on the increase, and it can affect the immune system as well.

How do you know if you're stressed? It's not always easy to tell, because one of the first things to go is your sense of judgement. But if you find you're getting irritable and short-tempered; lose your sense of humour, burst into tears at inappropriate moments, or start sleeping badly; if you realise that your eating habits have changed and you've doubled or halved your normal intake; if you've started smoking (again!) or find yourself drinking more than usual, the odds are you're suffering from stress. (See Chapter 11.)

DAVID'S STORY

'I had years of insomnia, made worse when my back gave up on me and I had to have an operation. Then followed months of chiropractic treatment, Alexander technique, you name it,

I tried it. But coincidentally, my tutor in the Alexander technique recommended a relaxation pose for me which has helped with the sleeplessness. I lie on the ground, on my side, with one leg across another, the knee raised to waist level. If I want, I have a blanket over me, and I listen to a relaxation tape. It certainly soothes my back, but it is also helping the insomnia, because I go to bed much less stressed each night. I know my stress is really caused by pain.'

Sleep problems are classically linked to stress. If you're overstressed, you're more likely to suffer from insomnia, and if you're not sleeping well, the quality of your life is almost certainly going to suffer as a result. The following auto-hypnosis technique is a highly effective stress-buster, and almost guaranteed to improve your chances of a good night's rest.

AUTO-HYPNOSIS

Imagine walking, slowly, down a set of twenty stairs. As you go down the stairs one by one, counting out 16, 15, 14 and so on, tell yourself you are descending into perfect peace and total relaxation. (It may sound corny, but it works.) Visualise the stairs if you can, in as much detail as possible.

Once you've reached the zone of tranquillity at the foot of the stairs, concentrate hard on staying there for a while. Repeat to yourself, 'This is a safe place. I'm safe here. It's a peaceful place. I am at peace.' Then begin to imagine a beautiful, sunlit scene. This should be one of your favourite places, which might be a warm and golden beach (remember Flora's story?) or a green woodland glade. Listen to the sounds of far-off surf, or faint birdsong. Feel the warmth of the sun on your skin, with the occasional soft breeze. (Audiotapes can be helpful.)

Finally, return to the space at the foot of the stairs. Slowly, counting as you go, climb the stairs until you get to the top stair. Open your eyes, but don't move just yet. Wait a few seconds, and then it's back to the real world – but you'll be carrying some of that deep relaxation with you. Your immune system (and your family) will notice the difference.

NB – Auto-hypnosis is a very powerful technique, and anyone considering using it should consult a reputable hypnotherapist. Alternatively, Robert Farago's book *Hypno Health* is one of the best and most accessible guides to the successful use of auto-hypnosis.

So there you have it. A de-stressing programme, a nutritional regime, a better sleep routine and an anti-smoking message. If you can manage those four, you'll be well on the way to better sleep.

Reference

Pharma Nord UK
  tel: 0800-591756

Hypno Health by Robert Farago (Vermilion)

CHAPTER 26

Acupuncture and acupressure

There are a fair number of the so-called alternative therapies, and if you have time and are sufficiently motivated, you could work your way through the list until you find one which works for you. Two of the most common are acupuncture and acupressure.

ACUPUNCTURE

Acupuncture can be an extremely effective remedy for insomnia. You may find that it takes several sessions to achieve very much of an effect, although some patients begin to feel a deep relaxation after or even during the first treatment. Its way of working cannot really be explained within the Western medical tradition, but practitioners say that it rebalances the body's energies.

The use of acupuncture in relieving pain is somewhat better understood, where it is thought to work by releasing endorphins, the body's own painkillers, in the brain; and also by blocking the nerves that carry the painful messages to the brain. In addition to relieving pain, acupuncture has also been found to be very helpful in treating withdrawal symptoms from sleeping pills or other addictive substances, including alcohol and heroin, and endorphins are thought to be involved here too.

The Chinese theory as to how acupuncture works is quite different, and is based on the concept that our health depends on a balanced and harmonious flow of life force. This life force, called *qi* or *chi*, is channelled through twelve main energy lines, or meridians. Each meridian is related to an organ, such as the heart, the liver and the lungs, and is named after that organ. Illness or disease has to do with an imbalance in life force – too much in one meridian, too little in another – and so the initial diagnosis relies heavily on checking the strength of the meridians. This is done by taking the patient's pulse at the wrist, which sounds quite orthodox; but where the Western medic finds one, the traditional Chinese acupuncturist finds no fewer than twelve pulses, one for each meridian. The acupuncturist will also take a medical history, and examine the patient's general appearance, before deciding on a course of treatment.

To rebalance the patient's *qi*, the acupuncturist must restore the correct energy flow in each meridian. Along each meridian lie hundreds of access sites, the acupuncture points, which can be used to turn the meridian's energy flow up or down. Treatment consists of selecting the appropriate acupuncture points, and manipulating them. Traditionally this was done with needles, but local percussion, pressure, or vibration all seem to be equally effective.

To most people, however, acupuncture means needles. In the standard procedure, tiny needles are inserted into the skin over the selected sites, and left there for 10 to 20 minutes at a time. The acupuncturist may roll the needles between finger and thumb occasionally, to increase the stimulation of the key sites; and some practitioners prefer not to use needles at all, but stimulate the key sites with little tablets of herbs, which are placed on the site, set alight and left to smoulder. This variant on the theme is called moxibustion. None of the above processes is particularly painful, although applying the needles or the heat to some sites may cause discomfort. Many find that with time, and as the course of treatment progresses, the degree of discomfort diminishes.

In the era of AIDS, we have all become very nervous of needles as a potential route of infection, but the acupuncturists are very aware of this, and either use strict sterilisation procedures approved by the DHSS or disposable needles.

There are a few appliances on the market which can be used on a D-I-Y basis. One of these is the Acuhealth, which has a dual function. It has sensors built into it which you can use to detect the key sites yourself; and then, once in place, it administers a small (and painless) electrical current which has the same effect on the site as a needle. I have used this device to reduce the pain of a torn muscle, and found it quite effective, but have not tried to use it for insomnia. However, the manufacturers supply an A to Z of the body, showing the meridian lines and main treatment sites, which you use as a guide to find your way to the approximate location of the site; the machine's finder mode does the rest. Acuhealth Ltd claim that their product can be used to treat insomnia, and at around £130, it could work out cheaper than a long course of acupuncture.

You might prefer to contact the British Acupuncture Association & Register for details of your local practitioner. The method doesn't work for everybody, but it's drug-free, and well worth trying.

ACUPRESSURE

For those who don't like the idea of needles, there is an alternative, namely acupressure. As its name suggests, this involves applying pressure, rather than needles, to the key points on the skin. Acupuncturists have long used certain points, located inside the wrist, to help patients achieve calm and improve the quality of their sleep. Green Farm produce a well-made preparation called Isocones. These are tiny, supple rubber cones, attached to adhesive tape which holds

them in place, and you apply one cone each night to your
own wrists. (If you're worried about how to find the right
spot, Green Farm include a wiring diagram which shows
how to site the cones correctly.)

You put the cones on each night before going to bed, and
they maintain a subtle, barely noticeable massaging action
over the acupressure point through the night. The interesting thing about this treatment is that it seems to have some
effect on most types of insomnia, whether it's difficulty in
falling asleep, broken sleep or early waking. The suppliers
recommend that the Isocones be worn for at least a month
before the full effects become apparent, but I noticed some
improvement (with regard to early waking) by the third
week.

Several small-scale studies found that many people using
Isocones who normally took sleeping tablets were able to
reduce their doses. About a third were able to come off their
medication altogether. However, if you have been taking
sleeping pills for a long time, it is not advisable to stop
suddenly. Instead, try combining Isocones with the tablets,
and see if you can get away with gradually reducing the
dose. Let your doctor know beforehand what you are planning to do, so if you do run into problems, he or she will be
able to help and advise.

References

Acuhealth Ltd
  Freepost (WD 4671)
  London
  W1E 4QZ

The British Acupuncture Association & Register
  34 Alderney Street
  London
  SW1V 3EU
  tel: 071-834 1012

Green Farm
  225 Putney Bridge Road
  London
  SW15 2PY
  tel: 081-874 1130

CHAPTER 27

Massage and oils

This is one of the most enjoyable ways of relaxing, and ironing out the mental and physical stresses which might otherwise keep you awake. Like acupuncture, the technique has been around for several thousand years, although it's only really taken off in Britain (famed for its reserve, and fear of touch) since the late seventies.

Some sorts of massage are more vigorous than others; sports massage, which goes for deep muscular manipulation, is fine for warming up before a squash game, and pretty good for relieving pain and stiffness afterwards, but for an easy descent into sleep you need something a little gentler.

Foot massage is a nice way to start, if you're not too ticklish. It works best with a little oil. If you decide to go out and buy a massage oil, go for one of the soothing, calming types, such as those with a lavender component. Neals Yard Apothecary and Robert Tisserand sell high quality oils; alternatively you can make up your own by adding 4 or 5 drops of the essential oil of lavender to 50 mls of a neutral oil base, such as avocado oil or cold-pressed grape seed oil, which are light, and well absorbed by the skin. Add a little wheatgerm oil to the mix, as this contains a high vitamin E content, which will keep the other oils from going rancid.

Don't make up more massage oil than you can use in 2 or 3 months, as the ingredients deteriorate with time, even with vitamin E, and store the mix in a dark glass bottle with an air-tight seal. Some aromatherapists recommend that the mix be kept in cool or cold storage, which could be at the back of the fridge. If you decide that this is the best place to keep your own special brand, label it clearly to make sure no one decides to use it for a fry-up; and remember to warm the oil between your hands before the massage begins.

This is especially important if you progress from the feet upwards to the neck and shoulders, another key site in de-stressing and relaxing. A sudden trickle of ice-cold oil between the shoulder blades will do nothing to help sleep problems, and could create another set of problems altogether.

If your partner is the one with the sleeping problem, he or she should lie back in a comfortable position against the pillows. Your place is halfway down the bed, and, sadly, because one of the nicest things about massage is savouring the other person's enjoyment, facing obliquely away from them. (This is because this position gives you the easiest access to the soles of your partner's feet.) Rest the lower leg on your lap, or across your thighs, so that it is slightly flexed, and the foot within easy reach.

Pour a little oil into the palm of one hand, and put the bottle down somewhere safe, such as a bedside table. Warm the oil between your hands, and then lightly smooth it over the main surfaces of the foot. There should be no friction or pulling against the skin. Then brace the heels of both hands on the upper surface of the foot, and knead the sole firmly, but not too vigorously, with stroking motions from the centre of the sole to the sides. Work your way up from the heel, through the arch and then the ball of the foot.

When you reach the toes, slow down. They require gentler and more individual treatment. Begin by flexing and then extending all the toes together, gently, two or three times. Then take the big toe with the finger and thumb of one hand, and run your index finger back and forth down in the gap between the toes, concentrating on the base of the toes where they join the foot. Do this several times in succession, and then repeat for all the other toes. Finish the routine by flexing and extending all the toes together, as before, and then give the sole of the foot one more going over. Finally, clasp the whole foot between both hands and squeeze it out, as if it were a cake of soap. Repeat 2 or 3 times.

If you're a real saint, and have strong hands, you could now repeat the entire procedure on your partner's other foot. If not, you could demand payment in kind before tackling the second foot. Alternatively, you could move upwards and concentrate on the neck and shoulders. This is where stress and strain usually accumulate, and untying the knots of muscle here can really help to smooth out the worries and resentments of the day.

One way of tackling this is to get the person who is to be massaged to sit at a table, leaning forward onto his or her folded arms. If you then stand behind and to one side, the whole neck and shoulder area is within reach. Alternatively, if the bed is sufficiently firm, you can easily use that as a massage table instead. If you lie your partner on his or her stomach, you'll find that the most comfortable working position is to sit astride him or her, below the waist. This position enables you to bear down with your body weight as and when you need to.

Whether you go for the table or the bed, the massage itself is the same. As with the feet, start by applying a thin film of massage oil over the working surface. There are many different massage styles, but my own preference is to start at the base of the spine, and work upwards. The following routine is pretty basic, but is a good way to start. You can make it increasingly elaborate and thorough as your stamina and imagination develop. It should take about ten minutes, and you'll find it as relaxing as the lucky recipient will.

Push the heels of both hands down from the buttocks into the small of the back, gently at first but increasing the pressure until you're using your entire body weight. (Listen to your partner. If at any step along the way, your partner is experiencing discomfort, ease up on the pressure.) Gradually work your way up along the spine, on a two steps forward and one back basis, until you reach the shoulderblades. This area needs a slightly different approach, as there are more moving parts. Now you'll have to use your thumbs, which should be aligned with the spine, with the fingers splayed out and pointing towards the shoulders. Push your thumbs along the lines of muscle which lie along the spine, until you come to the base of the neck; repeat several times, and then, still on the two steps forward and one back basis, begin to push from the spine out to the tips of the shoulders. Finally, get to work on the two ridges of muscle which connect the shoulder bone to the neck bone. Curl your fingers over the ridges, and squeeze them between fingers and thumbs – not too hard, or at this point your well-oiled partner is liable to jump, like a similarly squeezed orange pip, right out of the bed.

As you get more adventurous, the massage can be extended to include the buttocks, thighs, arms and head. You will soon find yourself looking forward to bedtime with an unfamiliar intensity, and although massage does not guarantee sleep, the relaxation and physical intimacy cannot help but make things better.

Massage is not only a venerable form of therapy, it's also extremely safe; but there are contra-indications. People with ultra-sensitive skins may react to certain essential oils, so test a patch of skin first before going the whole hog. Some skin problems such as serious acne, psoriasis and eczema are best left alone; areas of inflammation, and any open or infected sores and rashes should also be avoided. Finally, leg massage should not be given to anyone who has suffered from deep vein thrombosis, or who is bedridden, as it could dislodge blood clots with potentially dangerous results.

CAUTION: do not use essential oils neat, or take them internally. They are powerful medicines, and can cause skin irritation and other problems if they are not properly used. It is best to get advice from a qualified aromatherapist, or at the very least read through a good reference text to discover the basics, to avoid making potentially dangerous mistakes.

However, they are perfectly safe when used, in small quantities, in the bath. Ten or so drops of lavender oil mixed

well into the bath makes for a pungent, heady and relaxing
half-hour – if you can keep the rest of the family from
pounding on the door!

References

Neals Yard Apothecary
  1a Rossiter Road
  London
  SW12 9RY
  tel: 081-675 7144

Tisserand Aromatherapy Institute
  PO Box 746
  Hove
  East Sussex
  BN3 3XA

CHAPTER 28

Geopathic stress

An odd one this, but if you believe in crystal therapy and ley lines, then it's worth considering. The theory is that the quality of sleep may be influenced by force fields emanating from the earth, or that part of it under your bedroom; or by nearby powerlines, or even by bad plumbing. Incredible? Well, it's true that the earth's magnetic field can show local disturbances which are often associated with geological fractures. There is some evidence that underground rivers and deposits of certain metal ores can have a similar effect; and electric power lines are also known to generate force fields. But could all these things be bad for your sleep, or for your health, as some claim?

EMF AND MAGNETIC FIELDS

The problem is that the disturbances are actually of two sorts:

1. Electromagnetic fields (EMF), which are associated with high voltage power lines but in fact occur around nearly all electrical equipment
2. Purely magnetic fields, which emanate from the earth, or, for that matter, the magnets found in your loud-speakers and television set

There is a growing body of evidence linking EMF to ill health – 'Cell phones cause cancer!', read the scare headlines earlier this year – but just how much evidence is there? Sales of cell phones in America plummeted, and the Cellular Telecommunications Industry Association felt compelled to fund new studies; but looking back, the whole thing was sparked off by just four cases.

Last year two prominent US executives were stricken by brain cancer. Then in an unrelated and highly publicised lawsuit a Florida man, David Reynard, alleged that his wife's fatal brain cancer was caused by her cellular phone. Then folks remembered that Lee Atwater, the campaign strategist credited with winning the 1988 election for the Republicans, had also died of a brain tumour – and wasn't he, like the two executives, always walking around with a cell phone glued to his ear?

Given that thousands of people die of brain tumours every year, and had done so long before cell phones arrived on the scene, this might seem a tenuous connection, but the public was primed for it. The debate as to whether exposure to electromagnetic fields (EMF) might cause cancer had been raging for some time, and although the main focus was on power lines and visual display units, people were only too willing to believe that a small electromagnetic field, positioned close to the brain, might be harmful too.

The evidence linking EMF to health problems is patchy, but mounting. There are reports that people who work in an electrical profession have a 2.6 times greater risk of dying of myeloid leukaemia. There have been a number of findings of a fourfold increased risk of leukaemia in children living near overhead high tension lines. Reports of an increased incidence of miscarriage in VDU operators have been dismissed by the medical profession; but in the only study which divided VDUs into low, medium and high emitters, researchers found a clear correlation between intensity of exposure to EMF and the incidence of miscarriage.

However, it is not just VDUs and power lines. EMF is generated by *all* electrical appliances. Take hand-held radar guns: in the last year, dozens of State Troopers are reported to have been stricken with cancers of the eye, cheek or testicles (from holding radar guns between their legs). One recent study suggested that men who shave with electric razors are two to three times as likely to develop leukaemia as those who wet shave; and electric blankets, hair driers and televisions have all been called into question.

The problem with these findings is that the EMF generated by most appliances is simply too weak to affect human tissue by any well-known mechanism. It does not, for example, disrupt living cells or alter DNA in the way that ionising radiation does – but that isn't necessarily the end of the story. According to Nobel laureate Ilya Prigogine, 'The catastrophe in medicine is that we try to define the states of health and disease in terms of biochemistry, and forget the microphysics driving the tremendous physical machine which our body represents.'

Take a human cell – any cell. Every cell has a small charge, measured in millivolts, between its outside and its inside. An electrical engineer would call them micro-condensers. An adult has some 30,000 square feet of condenser surface in his or her body, with field charges of between 40 to 90 kilovolts/cm, constituting a complex electrical environment highly sensitive to EMF.

Some researchers have found a link between exposure to EMF and altered levels of the calcium ion, which carries a positive charge, inside the cell; and this in turn has been shown to lead to changes in cellular function, such as hormone production. It is early days yet, but this could be a mechanism by which exposure to EMF could cause ill health.

In the USA, various companies are already marketing devices claimed to smooth out 'electromagnetic turbulence'. Domestic and in-car models are available – but what other options are there? *Microwave News* and the *Townsend Letter*, a newsletter for doctors, recommend 'prudent avoidance'. If you can use an ordinary phone, do so. If mobility is needed, use a trunk-mounted car phone or two-piece cellular model that separates the hand-held receiver from the microwave transmitter. And as a rule of thumb, if you're close enough to touch a functioning electrical apparatus, you're too close.

EMF, then, is in the dock; but magnetism, however, has not so far come under serious suspicion. In fact, magnetism as a healing or malignant force has been under something of a cloud, in the scientific community at any rate, since Franz Mesmer's salon in revolutionary Paris was discredited by the leading savants of the day (who included the great scientists Benjamin Franklin and Antoine Lavoisier). They proved, to their own and most people's satisfaction, that Mesmer's magnetic force fields only acted through his patients' suggestibility.

However, if you prefer to believe in geopathic stress and its help in curing insomnia, then you could invest in one or two items of kit which have been designed to ward off this latter-day demonic force. Firstly, to see whether you have in fact been subjected to geopathic stress, you could invest in a Vegatest machine, much favoured by some practitioners, which measures something. If you prefer a more basic approach, look in your local alternative Yellow Pages under 'D', for Dowsers. Some of them will take the trouble to bring dowsing rods onto the premises; others, of a more sedentary disposition, prefer to wave a pendulum over the plans of your house. In either case, a wildly swinging or corkscrewing pendulum could spell trouble.

So what do you do? Some recommend a cork sheet. Placed under the mattress, it is supposed to absorb geopathic forces – but there are problems. It might shield you, if you're lying on top of it, but apparently it reflects the forces back downwards, which could be tough on the neighbours downstairs. And apparently it's not a permanent solution, because sooner or later (depending on such factors as the strength of the force field, the thickness of the cork and the credulity of the sleeper), it becomes saturated with geopathic stress and, it is claimed, loses its efficacy.

At this point you could buy a new one, or alternatively invest in a therapeutic crystal or two. Quartz is supposed to be good at soaking up the geopathic stresses, but you'll need a couple of lumps of the stuff – apparently a quartz watch won't do the trick, and nor will a quartz alarm clock! Then every morning, you must rinse the crystals under a cold tap, and the absorbed harmful energy, like the sins of our fathers, will be harmlessly washed away. Finally, for those who require even stronger medicine, there are a number of electronic gadgets on the market designed to soak up the harmful radiation, and your spare pounds.

Alternatively, you could move your bed, the plumbing, or your house into a less geopathically stressed area. Verdict: not proven, as they say in the Scottish courts, but none the less interesting. And if it works for you and you find a restful sleep, then there's no harm done.

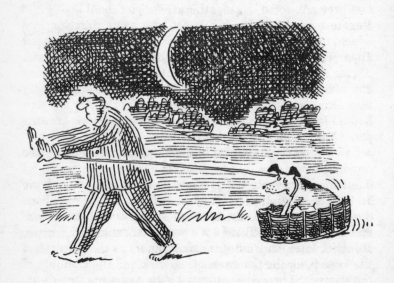

SLEEPWALKING

Sleep Diary

It's well worth while keeping a sleep diary, noting the main events of each day and the quality of the night's sleep. By keeping such a diary you may be able to see patterns emerging, and work out for yourself what factors might be contributing to the bad nights. And if things get worse, and you get to the stage of going to the doctor for help, the information in a sleep diary will be of considerable assistance in making an accurate diagnosis.

Part 1

To be filled out each day, by the patient:

1. Time of going to bed
2. How sleepy at time of going to bed?
3. How did you feel in bed?
4. Time taken to fall asleep (if known)
5. Time and duration of any waking periods during the night
6. How many hours' sleep?
7. How did you feel on waking?
8. Overall quality of sleep?
9. Sleeping pills taken
10. Other sleeping aids (herbal or other)
11. Other medication taken

Part 2

The first three questions can only be answered by the

insomniac's partner; the last three should be answered by both parties.

1. Does your partner stop breathing during the night? How often does this happen?
2. Does your partner snore, gasp or make choking sounds every night? How often does that happen?
3. Do your partner's legs twitch, jerk or kick during sleep? How often?
4. Have you noticed any recent change in the patient's moods?
5. Has the patient's consumption of alcohol, caffeine, nicotine or other drugs changed recently?
6. What do you think is the cause of the patient's difficulty in sleeping?

Useful Contacts

Pax
  4 Manorbrook
  Blackheath
  London
  SE3 9AW
  tel: 081-318 5026
  (anxiety, phobias, panic attacks)

Premenstrual Society
  PO Box 102
  London
  SE1 7ES
  (insomnia related to PMS)

National Debt Line
  318 Summer Lane
  Birmingham
  B19 3LR

Post-Traumatic Stress Disorder
  tel: 071-247 5164 Sundays helpline, 4.30–6.30 p.m.
  (for members of Armed Forces only)

Relaxation for Living
  168/170 Oatlands Drive
  Weybridge
  Surrey
  KT13 9ET
  tel: 0932-858355

MIND
22 Harley Street
London
W1N 2ED
tel: 071-637 0741

Be Not Anxious
16 Fairfield Road
Bosham
West Sussex
tel: 0643-572500

Association for Post Natal Illness
25 Jerdan Avenue
London
SW6 6RH
tel: 071-386 0868

Depressives Associated
PO Box 1022
London
SE1 7QB
tel: 081-760 0544

Alcoholics Anonymous
PO Box 1
Stonebow House
York
YO1 2NJ
tel: 071-352 3001

Council for Involuntary Tranquilliser Addiction (CITA)
Cavendish House
Brighton Road
Waterloo
Liverpool
L22 5NG
tel: 051-949 0102

British Society of Medical and Dental Hypnotists
8 Lonsdale Avenue
Giffnock
Glasgow
G46
(treat withdrawal symptoms by hypnosis)

Green Farm
225 Putney Bridge Road
London
SW15 2PY
tel: 081-874 1130

Medical Advisory Service
MAS is a registered charity, founded by nurses in 1986.
Its Helpline gives confidential help and advice to the
public on all aspects of health care and medical issues.
Run by nurses, the Helpline is staffed from Monday to
Friday, between 5 and 10 p.m. Tel: 081-994 9874.

Sleep Matters
A newsletter run by Monica Robb, for the Insomnia
Self-Help group. Contact Monica Robb on Thursdays at
10 Barley Mow Passage, Chiswick, London W4 4PH.
tel: 081-994 6477

National Institution of Medical Herbalists
Department H
9 Palace Gate
Exeter
EX1 1JA
tel: 0392-426022

Society of Homeopaths
2 Artizan Road
Northampton
NN1 4HU

tel: 0604-21400
(send SAE for a register of professional homeopaths,
information leaflets etc.)

Transcendental Meditation
FREEPOST
London
SW1P 4YY
tel: 0800-269303 (freephone)

Brain Machines

Brain machines is a generic term used to describe machines that train the brain to produce the alpha, theta and delta rhythms characteristic of the different stages of sleep. (See Chapter 1.) These machines have had a bad press, because in a few instances their use has reportedly triggered epileptic fits. However, the more up-to-date models are safe, because they do not operate at sufficiently high frequencies to cause any trouble.

The machines use various ways of training the brain to produce the desired frequency waves; pulsed lights are usually involved, and the more sophisticated models combine these with pulsed sound, and painless electrical shocks delivered to the body via modified electrodes known as TEMS units.

In the hands of a skilled operator, patients can be rapidly brought down from 15 cycles (beta waves, characteristic of the awake brain) to 12–14 cycles (alpha waves, associated with relaxation and drowsiness), and thence to theta and delta; by this stage, the patient is deeply asleep. After 2 or 3 sessions, people learn how to do this themselves, and many insomniacs have achieved complete cures this way. They simply wait until they're tucked up in bed, and then 'switch' their brains into sleep mode.

Unfortunately, there are no institutes that I know of in the UK that work to a sufficiently high standard; nor would I want to recommend any of the brain machines currently available here. The best clinic I know is in Rotterdam, and the hardened insomniac should certainly pay them a visit. It is called the Preventief Medisch Centrum.

The resident brain machine expert, William Barth, has had considerable success with even the most intractable of patients, and I recommend him unreservedly. And for those who might feel reluctant to pop across the North Sea to Rotterdam, there is an alternative – not quite as effective, perhaps, but certainly more convenient. It's an audio tape which uses some of the same principles as the Preventief Medisch Centrum method. Called the *Sound Sleep Tape*, it is available from Megabrain Sync., California. Prices have not yet been set, so write first and enquire.

References

Preventief Medisch Centrum
    Joost Banckertsplaats 24–29
    3012 HB Rotterdam
    The Netherlands
    tel: 010-3110 414 7633

Sound Sleep Tape audio tape
    Megabrain Sync.
    235 Bayview Street
    San Rafael
    California 94901
    USA

Index

Ability to concentrate and make decisions 3
Acupressure 128–9
Acupuncture 98, 100, 126–8
Adaptogens 82–3
Adolescents 46–8
Addresses, useful, *see* Useful addresses
Aerobics 87–8
Age/ageing
  change in sleep patterns 13–14
  insomnia and 41
  stress, ageing effects of 88
  varying sleep requirements 4–5
Aggression, testosterone levels and 92–3
Alarm clock, regular morning waking with a 66
Alcohol 28, 73–4, 93
Alfalfa juice 81
Allergens, exposure to during infancy 112
Allergies
  asthma 114–15
  hayfever 109–13
  sleep problems and 74–5
  see also Food allergies
Alternative medicine 99–100
Amounts of sleep required 4–5
Anxiety 29, 51–2
  technique to reduce 102–4
Aphrodisiacs, unlikely 95–6
Aromatherapy 35, 76, 131–2; *see also* Massage
Asthma 27, 48, 114–15
Audiotapes 76
Auto-hypnosis 124–5

Battlefield conditions, sleep studies 3
Bedding, house dust mites 114
Bedroom milieu 29–30
Bedtime
  food and drink 15, 74, 85–7
  recommended routine 64–5
  TV watching in bed 65
  winding down to 64
Benzodiazepines 58–9
Bereavement 40
Better sleep, steps towards 63–9
Biofeedback 99–100
Blood pressure, low 31
Blue light bulbs as sleep aid 76
Body clocks 67–8, 70–71
Brain machines 147–8
Brain tumours, cellular phones and 137
Breakfast
  energy-promoting recipe 79
  importance of 85
  liquid 82
British Association for Counselling 55, 57
Brostoff, Dr Jonathan 83

Caffeine 28, 35, 72, 107–8
Calcium 74, 108, 112
Case histories 10–11, 18, 33–4, 43–4, 53–4, 104, 105–6
Categories of insomnia 27–30
Causes of insomnia 2, 40–44
Celery as tranquilliser 75
Cellular phones, association with health problems 136–7

Central heating, house dust mites and 114
CFS, *see* Chronic Fatigue Syndrome
Chandra, Professor Ranjit 122
Childhood abuse, sleep problems associated with 28
Children
  night terrors 17, 20–21
  sleep problems 28–9, 45–6
Chinese meals 73
Chinese medicine 75–6, 77
Chromium deficiency 31
Chronic Fatigue Syndrome (CFS) 34–5
Circadian rhythm 67, 70
Co-enzyme Q (vitamin Q) 82
Coffee, *see* Caffeine
Cold viruses 116–19
  remedies 118–19
Concentration and decision-making 3
Conditioned insomnia 28–9
Council for Involuntary Tranquilliser Addiction (CITA) 9–10, 12
Counselling 53–5
Cramps 16, 27
Cystitis 86

Daylight, exposure to 64, 67–9, 94–5
Daytime napping 29, 64
Depression 28, 51–2, 70–71
Diary, recording sleep patterns in a 142
Dick, Dr Elliott 117
Diet
  to counter fatigue 35
  fruit 80, 81
  optimum nutrition 78–82
  vegetables 80–81
  for vitality 87
  yeast/sugar-free 84
Digestion problems 27
Digoxin 31
Doctor, consulting your 9–12, 50–53
Dowsing 139

Drinks, *see* Bedtime food and drink
Drugs 28, 72

Early waking 41–2
Elderly persons
  immune systems of 122
  sleep problems 41, 48–9
Electro-acupuncture 100, 101
Electromagnetic fields 136–9
Energy, diet for 82–3, 87
Enuresis 15
Essential oils
  cautionary note 134–5
  for massage 131–2
  sleep-inducing 76
Exercise
  aerobics 87–8
  as aid to sleep 64
  before breakfast 84
  effect on libido 93–4
  importance of 79
Extremes of sleep-deprivation 3

Fatigue and lack of energy 30, 79
Feedback loop as aid in panic attacks 109
Food allergies/intolerance 2, 74–5, 83–4, 115
Food cravings 83

Geopathic stress 136–40
Ginseng 82–3
GP, consulting your 9–12, 50–53
Green Energy, daily dose of 80–82
Growth Hormone, sleep-related release of 36–7
Guarana 83

Hayfever 109–13
Health
  cellular phones and 136–7
  sleep-deprivation and 37–8
  VDUs and 137
Heart attack, sleep apnoeacs 23–4
Herbs/herbal remedies 82–3, 75–6
  for childhood sleep problems 46
  for cold virus 118
  for loss of libido 96

Hiatus hernia 86
Homeopathic remedies 75, 76
Hormone Replacement Therapy,
    see HRT
Hormones, sex drive and 91–3
Horse chestnut blossom as
    aphrodisiac 95
House dust mites 114–15
HRT 41, 76, 91
Hypnosis 77, 99
Hypoglycaemia 75
    reactive 79

Ill health
    electromagnetic fields and 136–8
    sleep-denying illnesses 27
    sleep-deprivation as cause of 38
Immune system
    function of 120–21
    optimum nutrition essential to 122
    sleep-deprivation and 1–2
    smoking and 123
    stress and 123
    viruses and 117
INPUT 100
Insomnia
    causes 40–44
    chronic 39
    difficulty getting to sleep 40–41
    duration of 39–40
    early waking 41–2
    self-check 40–44
    short-term 39
    transient 39
    wakefulness 41
    see also Sleep
Iron deficiency 15, 31, 35
Irritability 3
Isocones 128–9

Jamaican dogwood 75, 76
Jet lag 70
Juices, vegetable and fruit 74, 81–2

Late-night eating or exercise 28, 85
Legs
    nocturnal cramps 16, 27
    restlessness 15–16, 74

Lettuce as tranquilliser 75
Libido, loss of 89–96
Life-shortening effect of insomnia
    37
Lifestyle, loss of libido and 93–4
Light
    benefits of 94–5
    effect on sleep-wake cycle 67–9,
        70–71
    exposure to 64, 67–9, 94–5
Light boxes 68–9
Light therapy 68

Magnesium 74, 108
Magnetic fields 139–40
Massage 99, 131–5
    contra-indications 134
    foot 131
    oils for 131–2, 134
    technique 132–4
ME, *see* Myalgic encephalitis
Meals, timing of 85–7
Medical problems as cause of
    insomnia 76
Meditation as anxiety-reducer
    102–4
Melatonin, function of 68, 70–71,
    94–5
Menopause 41, 76, 91
Mental pain control techniques 98
Mental relaxation at bedtime 65
Milky drinks 74
Mineral supplements 80–82, 87
    as aid in panic attacks 108
    calcium 74, 108, 112
    chromium 31
    for hayfever 112
    immune system and 122
    iron 15, 31, 35
    magnesium 74, 108
    zinc 96
Mitchel, Professor Peter 82
Moran, Dr John 93–4
Myalgic encephalitis (ME) 30, 34,
    35

Naps (daytime) 29, 64
Narcolepsy 17

Narcotics Anonymous 61, 62
Nasal allergies 109–13
Nasaleze 112, 113
Nicotine patches 72
Nightmares 14, 18–20
Night owls 67, 69
Night terrors 17, 20–21
Noise
   background, as sleep aid 66–7
   as cause of insomnia 30
Noradrenaline levels in the
   bloodstream 94, 95, 96
Northerly communities, incidence
   of sleep disturbance 71
Nutrition
   importance of, to immune system
      122
   optimum 78–82

Obstructive sleep apnoea syndrome
   see Sleep apnoea
Overweight, snoring and 22–3

Pain 97–8
   clinics 100–101
Panic attacks 105–8
   feedback loop 107
   treatment 107–8
Passwater, Dr Richard 117–18
Pharmacological causes of insomnia
   28
Phototherapy 68
Physical conditions causing
   insomnia 27
Physical relaxation, bedtime and 65
Physiological causes of insomnia 28
Pollen, hayfever sufferers 110–11
Post-traumatic stress disorder 28
Primary insomnia 52
Progressive relaxation techniques
   99
Prostate problems 13, 27, 86
Pseudo-insomnia 42
Psychiatric problems 29, 51–5
Psychological causes of insomnia
   28–9

Quartz, and geopathic stresses
   139–40

Reactive hypoglycaemia 79
Regular morning waking 66–7
Relaxation
   exercises in bed 65
   techniques 99
REM (Rapid Eye Movement) sleep
   7–8
Restless legs syndrome 15–16, 74
Rhinitis 110
Routine for bedtime 64–6

Seasonal Affective Disorder (SAD)
   67–9, 70–71, 94–5
Seasonal insomnia 109–13
Seasons, effect on libido 94–5
Self help for fatigue problems 35
Serotonin 74
Sex
   as aid to sleep 73
   benefits of 88, 89–90
   loss of libido 89–96
Shiftwork 16–17
Siberian ginseng 82–3
Skin cells, replacement of 37
Sleep
   core sleep 36
   different types of 5–8
   disorders 14–17
   deprivation, extremes of 3
   patterns, changes with age 13–14
   requirements 4–5
   slow-wave sleep 37
   stages of 6–8
   tiredness in spite of getting
      enough 42
Sleep apnoea 17, 23–4
   body builders and 26
   schoolchildren 25–6
   teenagers 48
Sleep diary 142
'Sleep hygiene' 29–30
Sleep labs 55–6
Sleep neurosis 28, 42–4
Sleep paralysis 14
Sleep tapes 76

Sleeping arrangements, insomnia and 2
Sleeping pills 9, 10–11, 40, 58–62
  coming off 60–62
  new developments 60
  side effects 59, 60
Sleepwalking 16
Smoking 28, 72, 123
Snoring 2, 14, 22–6
  age-related 22
  causes of 22–4
  devices to cure 25
  effect on partners 23
  overweight and 22–3
  sleep apnoea, *see that title*
  surgery to cure 25
  treatment for 24–5
Stages of sleep 6–8
Steroids, and sleep apnoea 26
Stress 2, 79
  de-stressing techniques 88
  effects of 123
  post-traumatic stress disorder 28
  remedies for 82–3
Sugar/yeast-free diet 84

Tea drinking to excess 15, 35, 107–8
Teenagers, sleep problems 46–8
Testosterone levels, sex drive and 91–3, 96
Thatcher, Margaret 4
Thyroid problems and loss of libido 91

Tinnitus 27
Tired All The Time Syndrome 30, 32–4
Tissue growth and repair during sleep 37
Traditional Chinese medicine 75–6
Tranquillisers 9–11
Transcendental meditation 77, 104
Tryptophan 74

Unwinding before bed 64
Useful addresses 12, 35, 57, 62, 69, 77, 84, 96, 101, 113, 125, 129–30, 135, 143–6

Valerian 75, 76, 77
VDUs, effects on health 137
Vegatest machine 139
Viruses, common cold 116–19
Vitamin supplements 35, 74, 80–82, 87, 96, 112, 117–18, 122

Wakefulness 41
Walking 79
Webster, Dr Stephen 88
Wheatgrass juice 81–2
Winter blues 67–9
Women as insomniacs 13, 38

Yeast/sugar-free diet 84

Zinc for hayfever 112
Zopiclone 60

Headline Health Kicks

Positive and practical advice to relieve persistent health problems.
Titles available include:

THE PRIME OF YOUR LIFE
Self help during menopause   Pamela Armstrong   £5.99   ☐

STOP COUNTING SHEEP
Self help for insomnia sufferers   Dr Paul Clayton   £5.99   ☐

AM I A MONSTER, OR IS THIS PMS?
Self help for PMS sufferers   Louise Roddon   £5.99   ☐

GET UP AND GO!
Self help for fatigue sufferers   Anne Woodham   £5.99   ☐

You can kick that problem!

All Headline books are available at your local bookshop or newsagent, or can be ordered direct from the publisher. Just tick the titles you want and fill in the form below. Prices and availability subject to change without notice.

Headline Book Publishing Ltd, Cash Sales Department, Bookpoint, 39 Milton Park, Abingdon, OXON, OX14 4TD, UK. If you have a credit card you may order by telephone – 0235 831700.

Please enclose a cheque or postal order made payable to Bookpoint Ltd to the value of the cover price and allow the following for postage and packing:

UK & BFPO: £1.00 for the first book, 50p for the second book and 30p for each additional book ordered up to a maximum charge of £3.00.

OVERSEAS & EIRE: £2.00 for the first book, £1.00 for the second book and 50p for each additional book.

Name..

Address...

....

....

If you would prefer to pay by credit card, please complete:
Please debit my Visa/Access/Diner's Card/American Express (delete as applicable) card no:

Signature..   Expiry date...................